GASTROINTESTINAL TNM CANCER STAGING BY ENDOSONOGRAPHY

GASTROINTESTINAL TNM CANCER STAGING BY ENDOSONOGRAPHY

T. Lok Tio, M.D., Ph.D.
Professor of Medicine
Division of Gastroenterology
Georgetown University Medical Center
Washington, DC

IGAKU-SHOIN   New York • Tokyo

Published and distributed by

IGAKU-SHOIN Medical Publishers, Inc.
One Madison Avenue, New York, New York 10010

IGAKU-SHOIN Ltd.,
5-24-3 Hongo, Bunkyo-ku, Tokyo 113-91.

Library of Congress Cataloging-in-Publication Data

Tio, T. L.
    Gastrointestinal TNM cancer staging by endosonography / T. Lok
Tio.
        p. cm.
    Includes bibliographical references and index.
    1. Gastrointestinal system—Cancer—Classification—Atlases.
2. Endoscopic ultrasonography. I. Title.
    [DNLM: 1. Gastrointestinal Neoplasms—ultrasonography—atlases.
2. Gastrointestinal Neoplasms—pathology—atlases. 3. Endoscopy,
Gastrointestinal—atlases. 4. Neoplasm Staging—atlases. WI 17
T594g 1995]
    RC280.D5T56   1995
    616.99′43307543—dc20
DNLM/DLC
for Library of Congress   94-21375
                                                              CIP

ISBN: 0-89640-267-3 (New York)
ISBN: 4-260-14267-4 (Tokyo)

Printed and bound in the U.S.A.
10 9 8 7 6 5 4 3 2 1

Dedication

This book is dedicated to my wife and children.

Acknowledgments

I would like to thank my former colleagues in the Department of Gastroenterology and Hepatology at the Academic Medical Center in Amsterdam, The Netherlands, and especially the head of the Department, Professor Guido Tytgat, who has extended continuing support toward the finishing of this book. Moreover, I greatly appreciate the assistance of Professor Dr. H.J. Houthoff, the former head of the Department of Pathology, who helped to select the pictures of corresponding histologic specimens. I would like, furthermore, to express my deepest appreciation to my former colleagues Dr. Kees Huibregtse, Dr. Joep F.W.M. Bartelsman, Dr. Christ J.J. Mulder, Dr. Dirk van Leeuwen, Dr. Eric Rauws and many others, particularly Dr. Jaques W.A.J. Reeders, the Head of the Department of Gastrointestinal Radiology and Hepatopancreatico-Biliary Imaging and to the Department of Surgery, particularly Prof. Dr. W.H. Brummelkamp, Prof. M.N. van der Heide, and Prof. Dr. Lykidakis. For assistance in preparing my publications I would like to express my thanks to my colleagues Dr. Oda Weijers, Dr. Paul R.A. Sars, Dr. Peter Paul L.O. Coene, Dr. Jan Udding, Dr. Lee-Hoei Sie, Dr. Nicola Kimmings, and Dr. Geert Luiken.

Finally, I would also like to express my sincere appreciation to my parents, who have always given me encouragement in this proejct, and to my wife Soan, our daughter Hong Xia, and our son Xiao Rui, without whose continuing support this work could not have been completed.

T. Lok Tio, M.D., Ph.D.

Preface

Over the past decade, clinical application of endosonography for staging and follow-up of diseases of the gastrointestinal tract has been increasing in many centers. This is primarily because dramatic improvements in image quality and instrument durability have combined with increasing knowledge of endosonographically important topographic anatomy and pathology to make endosonography the best available technique for accurately staging many gastrointestinal tumors.

The objective of the present work is to illustrate the endosonographic features of tumors of the digestive tract which have been classified according to the most recent edition of the *TNM Classification of Malignant Tumours* (P. Hermanek and L.H. Sobin, eds; Springer, 1987). The illustrations are accompanied by detailed legends and explanatory text. Throughout the work, the endosonographic findings obtained with a radial scanning echoprobe have been compared with those of endoscopy, x-ray examination, and the histology of resected specimens. It is hoped that this atlas will prove valuable to internists, gastroenterologists, surgeons, radiologists, and other physicians who diagnose and treat gastrointestinal tumors. Clinical TNM staging of carcinoma of the digestive tract will hopefully become the standard diagnostic procedure in the clinical management of cancer patients.

T. Lok Tio, M.D., Ph.D.

Contents

INTRODUCTION

Since its original development by Denoix between 1943 and 1952, several revisions of the TNM system have been published (T, extent of primary tumor; N, presence/absence and extent of regional lymph node metastasis; M, presence/absence of distant metastasis). The classification of tumors on the basis of the anatomical extent of disease is determined clinically (nonsurgical) and histopathologically (postsurgical).[1-3] The pathological TNM classification (pTNM) is widely used for classification of carcinomas of the digestive tract; clinical TNM classification (cTNM), however, has been less well established. Various imaging techniques are used for staging. Evidence obtained from such special diagnostic means as ultrasonography is defined as C2, that from surgery as C3, histological examination of resected specimens as C4, and autopsy as C5. Recently, the depth of tumor infiltration has become the criterion for clinical classification, replacing the factors of size, circumferential involvement, and topographic distribution.[1,2] The correlation between clinical and pathological classifications is becoming increasingly important in establishing clinical TNM staging. Pancreatic and bile duct carcinoma were first included in the most recent (1987) TNM version. Achieving uniformity in classifying carcinomas of the digestive tract is now becoming a reality in clinical application.

Endosonography (EUS) was developed to improve ultrasound images by directly imaging the target lesion via the digestive tract with a high-frequency ultrasound probe.[4-12] A previously unknown, high-quality resolution can be obtained on the basis of real-time properties, 360° radial scanner of high frequency, and high resolution of ultrasound equipment. This imaging system permits accuracy in the staging of carcinoma of the digestive tract through detailed topographic anatomical images, high-quality resolution, and close correlation of EUS findings on the depth of gastrointestinal tumor infiltration with the histology of resected specimens. The wall of the digestive tract is imaged as a five-layer ultrasonographic architecture using a switchable 7.5 or 12 MHz EUS instrument, which shows a close correlation with the macroanatomy. This interpretation of the wall is generally accepted.[5,6,13,14] The interfaces between the various layers have been thoroughly studied, and the interpretation of individual layers is now established.[15] EUS has proven the most suitable modality for imaging the intestinal wall architecture. Moreover, a new dimension in staging biliopancreatic carcinoma can be obtained by the ability to visualize both parenchymal and ductular abnormalities and their adjacent lymph nodes.[5,6,9,10]

The most important advantage of EUS lies in the ability it affords to detect the early stages of disease and to stage nonresectable carcinomas. Detecting the disease at an early stage is essential for selecting patients who might benefit from surgery, endoscopic resection or laser photocoagulation, and determination of resectability is important to avoid unnecessary exploratory surgery. The ideal imaging technique would distinguish potentially curable from incurable stages of disease. Moreover, follow-up after surgical or nonsurgical treatment (laser, irradiation, chemotherapy) may become essential in detecting local recurrence, residual tumors, and the response to therapy. Response and nonresponse can be objectively imaged and documented. This information is important for interdisciplinary collaboration in planning the strategy of treatment. I therefore believe that EUS will become the standard diagnostic imaging technique for staging carcinomas of the digestive tract on the basis of the TNM classification.

The terms used in describing EUS images correspond to those of transcutaneous ultrasonography. *Hyperechoic* refers to a strongly echogenic pattern. *Hypoechoic* means weakly echogenic, that is, a pattern of low echogenicity density. And *anechoic* refers to the lack of echogenic pattern, caused by the total reflection of ultrasound and appearing as "black" structure on the image. Recently, echogenicity can be objectively measured by using a EUM20 observation unit. In this manner, subjective judgment can be replaced by an imaging modality.

PRIMARY TUMORS OF THE UPPER DIGESTIVE TRACT

Clinically and technically, EUS is subdivided into that of the upper and that of the lower digestive tract. The former consists of EUS of the esophagus, stomach, pancreas, papilla of Vater, distal and proximal extrahepatic bile ducts, and gallbladder; the liver is excluded because of the limited depth of ultrasound penetration. Lower intestinal EUS comprises that of the rectum and suprarectal colonic segments; these are described in Chapter 3.

Instruments

At present, there are three types of ultrasound instruments:

> Echoendoscope (fiberoptic or videoechoendoscope) consisting of a side or forward viewing endoscope;
> Nonoptic flexible ultrasound instrument (flexible or rigid);
> Endoscopic-guided catheter echoprobe (radial or linear array).

Since 1983, we have been using an Olympus prototype fiberoptic echoendoscope (EUM1) for upper digestive EUS or the now commercially available, modified model (EUM2).[5] The length of the rigid tip is 45 mm (EUM1) or 42 mm (EUM2). The frequency of the ultrasound wave is 7.5 MHz, the penetration depth is approximately 10 cm, and the theoretical axial resolution is 0.2 mm. Axial resolution is defined in terms of the ability to distinguish the two nearest points within a transmitted wave of the ultrasound beam. The resolution depends on the wave length of the ultrasound and the capability of the transducer. Recently we have been using an Olympus prototype instrument with a frequency of 10 MHz, a penetration depth of approximately 5 cm, and an axial resolution of 0.15 mm. The newest commercially available model (EUM3) emits an adjustable frequency of 7.5 MHz or 12 MHz—the latest is of clinical advantage for lesions adjacent to or in the digestive tract—and has a biopsy channel for EUS-guided cytological puncture and endoscopic biopsy.[6,9] The penetration depth of the 12-MHz ultrasound beam is 3 cm, and the axial resolution is approximately 0.12 mm. The penetration depth of ultrasound decreases with the increase in frequency. Recently an Olympus prototype videoechoendoscope (VUM2) emitting an ultrasound frequency of 7.5 MHz has become available. The transducer is approximately 12 mm long and has an outer diameter of 10 mm; the diameter of the side-viewing endoscope is 13 mm. The quality of its endoscopic images is superior to those of the fiberoptic instrument, and the ultrasound images are comparable to those of the standard fiberoptic echoendoscope.

The most recently developed fiberoptic echoendoscope (XJFUM3) has a smaller echoprobe (diameter 10 mm, length 42 mm) and a bridge for positioning the biopsy forceps, aspiration cytology needle, and even a catheter for cannulation of Vater's papilla. This may enable simultaneous EUS and endoscopic retrograde cholangiopancreatography (ERCP) as well as therapeutic puncture during EUS, for example, the drainage of pancreatic pseudocysts, sclerotherapy, and even biliary stenting. This, however, requires adequate disinfection procedure of the instrumental channel. In the case of severe esophageal stenosis which cannot be passed with an echoendoscope, a flexible small-caliber nonoptic Aloka prototype instrument with a length of 65 cm is available; the transducer is 30 mm long and has an outer diameter of 10 mm. This instrument has not been further developed. A similar small-caliber flexible nonoptic Olympus prototype has become available which can be inserted via a flexible guide wire. This must be placed using a regular gastroscope before EUS into and beyond the stenotic area.[12]

A small catheter Olympus prototype echoprobe is available which can be passed through the large biopsy channel of a gastroscope (GIF-T10). The echoprobe is 3 mm in diameter, and the rigid tip is 15 mm long; the frequency of this mechanically rotating radial echoprobe is 7.0 MHz. Images obtained are comparable in quality to those from the previously described instruments; however, the resolution is lower than that of the standard EUS instruments because of the very small size of the transducer. In the near future, a small balloon attached at the transducer for improving ultrasound images will become necessary.

Table 1 summarizes the technical data of the instruments used in the present series of patients.

Recently, a color Doppler echoendoscope has also become available, which may become important in evaluating vascular abnormalities.

Investigation Techniques

The echoendoscope is inserted like any other endoscope after local oropharyngeal anesthesia and intravenous sedation with diazepam (Valium) or midazolam (Dormicum). Intravenous sedation is necessary because of discomfort to the patient when introducing the rigid tip and insufflating the balloon with water or filling the gastroduodenal lumen with water. The instrument must be introduced blindly into the esophagus because the lateral-viewing optics do not allow endoscopic visualization of the esophagus. In the absence of severe stenosis, the endoscope is inserted into the stomach and duodenum for visualizing the desired structures. After the balloon attached at the echoprobe and bowel is filled with degassed water, the instrument is gently withdrawn until the target lesion is visualized ultrasonographically. Freezing ultrasound images is essential for photographic documentation, and various sections are necessary for assessment of the maximal extent of carcinoma. Real-time ultrasound images, however, are the most essential part of EUS interpretation. Lymph nodes along the known anatomical site must be identified and staged.

For practical reasons, description of the instruments and the technique of investigation for colorectal carcinomas has been included in the chapter on such carcinomas (see page 28). Anatomical orientation of EUS images is illustrated separately.

Esophagus

Technique

To visualize the lymph nodes at the celiac trunk, the echoendoscope is introduced into the stomach paracardially and along its lesser curvature. Images such as cross-sectional scans of computed tomography (CT) are used for standardization of EUS investigation. Longitudinal and oblique sections are obtained by maneuvering the echoprobe using the descending aorta as a landmark or by placing the liver and the spleen in the longitudinal or oblique position as in transcutaneous abdominal ultrasound. The echoendoscope is withdrawn gradually until the infiltrating abnormality with adjacent lymph nodes is clearly visualized by ultrasound. The longitu-

Table 1. Technical Data of Various Olympus Echoendoscopes

Echoendoscope	GIF-EUM2	GIF-EUM3	VU M2 (video)	XIF-UM3	Endoscopic-catheter echoprobe
Endoscope	Side-viewing gastroscope	Side-viewing duodenoscope	Side-viewing gastroscope	Side-viewing gastroscope	Forward-viewing (GIF-T10/GIF20)
Echoprobe	Mechanical sector or radial scanning (180°)	Mechanical sector or radial scanning (180° or 360°)	Mechanical sector or radial scanning (180° or 360°)	Mechanical sector or radial scanning (180° or 360°)	Catheter echoprobe (radial scanning 180° or 360°)
Length (mm)	42	42	44	42	In total 14 mm with the cathether
Diameter (mm)	13	13	10.4	10	3
Frequency (MHz)	7.5	7.5/12*	7.5	7.5	7
Depth of penetration (cm)	10	10/3	10	10	3
Axial resolution (mm)	0.2	0.2/0.12	0.2	0.2	Not known presently (prototype)
EUS-guided puncture/biopsy	No	Yes	No	A bridge (elevator) for sonography-guided puncture or biopsy	No

* Switchable frequency.

dinal extent of tumor can be assessed endoscopically by measuring the distance between the teeth and both the distal and proximal edges of the abnormal area. Usually we use the information gathered by previous routine gastroscopy with a forward-viewing gastroscope. During withdrawal from the cervical esophagus, water should be removed from the balloon in order not to compress the trachea, thus causing discomfort to the patient. In the case of severe stenosis that cannot be passed with echoendoscope, a flexible Aloka instrument of smaller caliber is available which can be introduced gently into the stomach past the stenotic area to image the full extent of tumor infiltration and lymph node involvement. The nomenclature from the Japanese classification of regional lymph nodes can be incorporated to facilitate defining the anatomical site of lymph nodes. In Western countries, however, such classification may not be widely used because of its rather complicated system. An alternative approach would be an accurate description of the pathological lymph node related to the tumor—the distance between the proximal or distal edge of the tumor and the lymph node—or use of the common nomenclature of lymph nodes, e.g., carinal, paracardial, retrocardiac, etc. EUS should not be performed immediately after endoscopic dilatation because of the high risk of perforation after dilatation. Recently we have been using the catheter echoprobe and have introduced it through the biopsy channel of a large-caliber gastroscope into the narrow filiform stenosis under endoscopic (optic) guidance. The anatomical site of the carcinoma, i.e., the distance between the teeth and the carcinoma, can be identified using the aorta, left atrium, and left lobe of the liver as landmarks. In the proximal esophagus, the trachea, carotid arteries, jugular veins, aorta, and thyroid gland are the most important landmarks.

Interpretation

The interpretation of the structure of the wall of the digestive tract and the nearby lymph nodes is based on results obtained through prior detailed examination of resection specimens and autopsy materials.[4,5,13] In essence, EUS visualizes a five-layer structure: The first hyperechoic and second hypoechoic structures correspond to the bordering echo and the mucosa. The third hyperechoic structure corresponds to the submucosa and the interface echo. The fourth hypoechoic structure corresponds to the muscularis propria. The fifth hyperechoic structure corresponds to the adventitia and the interface echo. Interface echoes between different media should be taken into consideration when comparing the results of EUS with the histological findings. The gastrointestinal wall appears thicker upon EUS than upon histology.[14] The thickness of the interface echo appears to correlate with the axial resolution of the transducer.

For histological (pathological) classification of carcinoma the most recent version of the TNM (pTNM) system is used. This combines evaluations of the T, N, and M criteria. For the esophagus, the depth of tumor infiltration (T) is categorized into four groups, involvement of regional lymph node metastases (N) into two, and involvement of distant metastases (M) likewise into two groups. Patterns that may be expected to entail similar prognosis are grouped into stages. EUS-based stages may show discrepancies to pathological stages as a result of overstaging or understaging of tumor infiltration or of false-positive or false-negative diagnosis of regional or distant metastasis. The categories for each criterion and the stages formed through their combination are as follows:

T: Primary tumor
T1:   Tumor invading lamina propria or submucosa
T2:   Tumor invading muscularis propria
T3:   Tumor invading adventitia
T4:   Tumor invading adjacent structures
    Tx: Primary tumor cannot be assessed.

N: Regional lymph nodes
N0:   No regional lymph node metastasis (excluding celiac lymph nodes)
N1:   Regional lymph node metastasis (excluding celiac lymph nodes)
    Nx: Regional lymph nodes cannot be assessed.

M: Distant metastasis
M0:   No distant metastasis
M1:   Distant metastasis: hepatic metastasis, peritoneal dissemination, or lymph node metastasis at the celiac trunk (pleural and peritoneal dissemination being rare)
    Mx: Distant metastasis cannot be assessed.

Stage grouping
Stage I: T1 N0 M0
Stage IIA: T2 N0 M0, T3 N0 M0
Stage IIB: T1 N1 M0, T2 N1 M0
Stage III: T3 N1 M0, T4 N0 M0, T4 N1 M0
Stage IV: Any T, any N M1

EUS classification of the depth of tumor infiltration is made according to pathological TNM (pTNM):

EUS-T1:   Hypoechoic tumor localized in the first (mucosa type), second, or third echo layer (submucosa type)

EUS-T2:   Hypoechoic tumor in the first three echo layers, extending into the fourth layer

EUS-T3:   Hypoechoic transmural tumor (first, second, third, and fourth structures), with penetration into the fifth layer

EUS-T4:   Hypoechoic transmural tumor with penetration into adjacent structures such as pericardium, descending aorta, tracheobronchial tree, diaphragm (curva diaphragmatica), or liver. Accurate definition of penetration into adjacent structures should be described as follows: no clear demarcation between the tumor and the adjacent organ irregularities of the organ contour, e.g., aorta, jugular vein, tracheobronchial tree, etc.

Criteria for assessing lymph node metastases are used as follows. Lymph nodes with hypoechoic pattern and clearly delineated boundaries are suspect for malignancy. Direct extension of mural abnormalities into adjacent lymph nodes is highly suspect for malignancy. Lymph nodes with a hyperechoic pattern and indistinctly demarcated boundaries are indicative of nonmalignancy, benign disease, or benign tissue.[15,16]

EUS is accurate in assessing the depth of tumor infiltration because of its ability to image the individual layers of the digestive tract wall. A close correlation between EUS findings and the histology of resected specimens can be demonstrated.[6,8] Obtaining various sections is crucial for assessing the maximal depth and the extent of carcinomatous infiltration. This has proven to be essential for comparing the clinical (c) T category with the highest pathological (p) T category, which is the most relevant criterion for tumor classification. The early stage of disease can be distinguished from advanced stages on the basis of the depth of tumor infiltration. Destruction of the esophageal wall architecture after irradiation or as the result of inflammatory changes beyond those of an ulcerative lesion may suggest a more advanced stage of carcinoma on ultrasound. This may lead to overstaging.[17] Early esophageal carcinoma is defined as a T1 carcinoma without evidence of lymph node involvement. In contrast, an early gastric carcinoma defined as a carcinoma limited to the mucosa and submucosa (T1) may be associated with regional lymph node metastases. A modified definition of early esophageal carcinoma, based on Chinese and Japanese experiences, may point to the highly malignant nature of the disease. Understaging of carcinomatous infiltration may occur as the result of a severe stenosis that cannot be passed with the EUS instrument. In such cases, the maximal extent of infiltration beyond the stenotic area cannot be assessed.

The results of EUS in preoperative assessment of the depth of tumor infiltration have been published elsewhere.[6] In our series (N = 74) the accuracy of EUS in the evaluation of T1 carcinoma was 80%, in T2 89%, in T3 83%, and in T4 78%. The overall accuracy was 83%.

The number of lymph nodes found in resected specimens varies. In our series, the number varied from 1 to 58 with an average of 7. The metastasis rate was approximately 37%. EUS is more accurate in diagnosing metastatic lymph node involvement than nonmetastatic lymph nodes. A pathognomonic echo pattern for defining malignant lymph node involvement is one showing direct penetration of the mural abnormality into adjacent lymph nodes, for example, granulomatous inflammation; sarcoidosis, however, may simulate the presence of malignancy. The overall accuracy of EUS in diagnosing regional lymph nodes was 85%. Sensitivity was 94% and specificity 56%; the positive predictive value was 83% and the negative predictive value 94%. When lymph nodes are excluded that are not stageable by EUS (EUS-Nx), the accuracy was 85%. In the evaluation of distant metastasis EUS is accurate for staging metastases in the celiac lymph nodes but less accurate for those in the liver or peritoneum because of the limited penetration depth of ultrasound. Moreover, severe luminal stenosis due to cancerous infiltration that cannot be passed with the instrument must be excluded from evaluation. In such cases, transcutaneous abdominal ultrasound or CT often proves helpful.

In stage grouping, the accuracy of EUS is often attenuated due to incorrect diagnosis of the T or M category. Since stage grouping is a combination of these three categories, an incorrect diagnosis in any of the three may lead to erroneous assignment to a stage group. In our series, the incidence of nonstageable distant metastasis (EUS-Mx) was relatively high due to severe stenosis.

The incidence of lymph node metastasis increases with the depth of tumor infiltration. The frequency of metastases increases rapidly from T1 to T2 carcinoma. This may explain the poor prognosis of the advanced stage of the disease.

CT has been reported to be accurate in the staging of esophageal carcinoma. Recent reports, however, indicate the accuracy of CT to vary from 39% to 100%. The new (1987) TNM classification has not been used for staging esophageal carcinoma by CT. We carried out a study of the preoperative TNM classification of esophageal carcinoma by EUS and CT to assess the accuracy and the limitations of each imaging technique. For CT staging, pT1 and pT2 carcinoma were grouped together because CT is not able to image the muscularis propria, making the distinction between these two groups impossible. Criteria for the assessment of the depth of tumor infiltration with CT were as follows:[6]

CT-T2 (pT1 + pT2):	Wall thickness of approximately 10 mm
CT-T3 (pT3):	Wall thickness of more than 10 mm without evidence of invasion into adjacent structures.
CT-T4 (pT4):	Wall thickness of more than 10 mm with evidence of invasion into adjacent structures.

In assessing the depth of tumor infiltration, EUS proves more accurate than CT in diagnosing the early stages (T1 and T2) and nonresectability (T4) of the disease. In diagnosing the less advanced stage of carcinoma (T3) the two techniques are equally accurate. This overall superiority of EUS is of utmost importance for the clinical management of patients. Early stages of the disease should be treated surgically whenever possible, whereas patients with an advanced stage of disease (nonresectable) should not undergo surgery due to the poor long-term prognosis. Resectability should be defined by noninvasive, preoperative staging instead of exploratory surgery.

EUS is more accurate in diagnosing metastatic involvement of regional lymph nodes, however, CT is more accurate in determining the presence of (nonmetastatic) benign lymph nodes. Since the diagnosis of lymph node metastasis is essential for the selection of patients for surgery, the superiority of EUS in diagnosing lymph node metastasis makes it clinically more relevant. As noted above, because of the limited penetration depth of ultrasound, CT is more accurate in diagnosing liver metastasis. In the diagnosis of celiac lymph node metastasis, CT is also more accurate in cases of severe stenotic carcinoma. On the other hand, however, EUS is superior in cases of less severe stenotic carcinoma. EUS is accurate for staging esophageal carcinomas regardless of their localization, but CT is not as reliable for staging carcinoma of the gastroesophageal junction as for that of the esophagus.

Neither EUS nor CT is always accurate in disease staging because a single incorrect diagnosis of the T, N, or M category may lead to an incorrect stage assessment. When those cases that are not stageable by EUS (EUS-Tx, EUS-Nx, EUS-Mx) are excluded, EUS is more accurate than CT.

Difficulty in Diagnosing T4 of Air-Containing Organs and Bony Structures

The difficulty in diagnosing T4 esophageal cancer, invading the tracheobronchial tree, the pleural cavity, and the vertebral spine has been recognized by many endosonographers. The trachea and the bronchus are visualized as a hyperechoic pattern associated with repeat echos (reverberation phenomenon). The trachea is located ventrally to the esophagus, whereas the location and the shape of the bronchus are variable, depending on its topographic anatomical relation with the esophagus. Tumor invasion into the trachea and the bronchus is visualized as a hypoechoic tumor mass, which shows a close proximity to the hyperechoic trachea or bronchus. The border between the tumor and the trachea or the bronchus cannot be recognized anymore because the tumor is invading the posterior wall of the tracheobronchial system. Bronchoscopy may be negative, resembling the similarity with submucosal tumors in the GI tract. Transbronchial aspiration cytology should be attempted to achieve a tissue diagnosis. Tumor invasion beyond the trachea or the bronchus or both is less complicated for endosonographers and bronchoscopists. On EUS such a tumor is seen as a hypoechoic mass penetrating into the anterior wall of the trachea or bronchus. On bronchoscopy a tumor mass protruding into the tracheobronchial lumen may be observed. Tumor invasion into the pleural cavity is difficult to diagnose by EUS because the air-containing lungs produce a lot of artifact. In my own experience such a diagnosis can be suggested by the presence of pleural effusion and the tumor penetrating into the adjacent fluid–pleura surface. Clinically, a positive diagnosis of transcutaneous pleural puncture is a confirmation of widespread disease and surgery is a contraindication. Tumor invasion into the vertebral spine is visualized as a hypoechoic tumor mass penetrating into the surface of hyperechoic arched pattern of the vertebra. To avoid overstaging, at least one-third of the circumference of the arched hyperechoic vertebra should be involved by the tumor. The surgeon usually states that the tumor is fixed to the vertebral spine or that if the tumor had been removed, the histology would reveal a nonradical resection.

Despite the difficulties mentioned, the overall accuracy gathered from seven major centers shows similar results to those we have experienced: the accuracies for tumor staging and for regional metastases were 80% and 75%, respectively.[18] This may reflect the relatively less complicated anatomic route—the tubelike structure of the esophagus—and the clear demarcation between each category of tumor and lymph node, which can be almost uniformly done by various investigators.

Comments

EUS is the most reliable imaging technique in the preoperative TNM classification of esophageal carcinoma. Thus, cTNM can be applied with EUS and generally corresponds to pTNM. For this reason, clinical application of the TNM classification will likely become the trend in the near future. In our prospective study, EUS proved more accurate than CT because of the ability to image the individual layers of the wall of the digestive tract and adjacent lymph node involvement even when the diameter was less than 5 mm. Moreover, the real-time properties of ultrasound and the ability to achieve various cross-sections by EUS makes this form of imaging superior to the static character and single-orientation sections of CT. One of the most important advantages of EUS over CT is the tissue diagnosis obtained by EUS-guided aspiration cytology or biopsy. Recently, other authors have confirmed our findings that EUS is superior to CT in staging tumor categories and regional lymph nodes. The availability of small-caliber ultrasound instruments, particularly the catheter echoprobe, during routine endoscopy can be expected to make EUS the most exciting diagnostic procedure for gastroenterologists who wish to stage esophageal carcinoma during early consultation procedures. In the near future, the transformation of side-view optics into forward-viewing instruments with a remarkable reduction in the outer diameter of the echoprobe will be necessary for performing simultaneous endoscopic and ultrasound investigations in a single procedure.

Case Report

A 63-year-old man suffering from angina pectoris was referred to a gastroenterologist due to abdominal discomfort. Endoscopy revealed a small ulcerative lesion in the distal esophagus. The biopsy was positive for carcinoma. EUS revealed a small intrasubmucosal hypoechoic tumor with no evidence of regional lymph node involvement or distant metastases (T1N0M0) (Figure 10). After consultation with a cardiologist no contraindication for surgery was found. The histology of the resected specimen confirmed the EUS findings. The patient was discharged from hospital in good condition 2 weeks after surgery.

Case Report

A 45-year-old woman was referred to a gastroenterologist because of dysphagia. Endoscopy revealed a carcinoma in the upper third of the esophagus, and CT showed a concentric thickening of the esophageal wall. EUS showed an extensive transmural infiltration with penetration into the dorsal wall of the trachea approximately 5 cm under the sphincter of the esophagus. Deep transmural infiltration in the contralateral side adjacent to the vertebra was also found. Multiple regional lymph nodes were present (T4N1Mx). Intraluminal radiotherapy with additional external radiotherapy was preferred over surgery because of the nonresectable stage of the disease. The patient is still in good condition 12 months after treatment.

Stomach

Technique

The technique of EUS investigation resembles that of gastroscopy. The lesion should first be found endoscopically; the echoprobe is then positioned as closely as possible to the target lesion. The space between the echoprobe and the lesion must be filled with water to achieve a clear ultrasound image (acoustic coupling). The gastric lumen or the balloon attached at the transducer is filled with water; the method of the water-filled stomach is more suitable than the water-filled balloon to visualizing the intraluminal extent and configuration of the lesion, for the gross appearance of carcinomas seen by endoscopy can then be correlated with the ultrasound image. However, lesions that cannot be coated with water should be investigated with the balloon method, for example, those of the cardia, pylorus, and anterior wall of the stomach. To visualize the infra- and suprapyloric lymph nodes, the echoprobe should be placed in the pylorus. Lymph nodes adjacent to the major blood vessels should be identified using the corresponding blood vessels as landmarks, for example, the celiac trunk, splenic artery, hepatic artery, superior mesenteric artery, portal vein, and splenic hilum. In visualizing lymph nodes along the lesser curvature of the stomach, the clinician can use the left lobe of the liver as a landmark. By slowly withdrawing the echoprobe into the esophagogastric junction, pericardial lymph nodes can readily be found. Thereafter, periesophageal lymph nodes should be identified. The Japanese nomenclature of lymph nodes can be incorporated to give exact information for the surgeon in performing radical lymph node dissection.

Interpretation

The interpretation of the gastric wall images is as with that of any other gastrointestinal wall. The serosa cannot be distinguished from the subserosal layer except when intraperitoneal ascites is present. In such cases, the serosal layer appears as a hyperechoic pattern directly adjacent to the ascites fluid. The interface echo between ascites and the serosa, however, should be taken into consideration. Thus, the serosal layer appears thickened on ultrasound compared with the real thickness demonstrated at histology.

T: Primary tumor
T1:   Tumor invading lamina propria or submucosa
T2:   Tumor invading muscularis propria or subserosa
T3:   Tumor invading serosa
T4:   Tumor invading adjacent structures
    Tx: Primary tumor cannot be assessed.

N: Regional lymph nodes
N0:   No regional lymph node metastasis
N1:   Metastasis in perigastric lymph node(s) within 3 cm of the edge of the tumor
N2:   Metastasis in perigastric lymph node(s) more than 3 cm from the edge of the primary tumor or in lymph nodes along with left gastric, common hepatic, mesenteric, splenic, or celiac arteries
    Nx: Regional lymph nodes cannot be assessed.

M: Distant metastasis
M0:   No distant metastasis
M1:   Distant metastasis: hepatic metastasis, peritoneal dissemination
    Mx: Distant metastasis cannot be assessed.

Stage grouping
Stage IA: T1 N0 M0
Stage IB: T1 N1 M0, T2 N0 M0

Stage II: T1 N2 M0, T2 N1 M0, T3 N0 M0
Stage IIIA: T2 N2 M0, T3 N1 M0, T4 N0 M0
Stage IIIB: T3 N2 M0, T4 N1 M0
Stage IV: T4 N2 M0, any T, any N M1

Early gastric carcinoma (T1) appears as a circumscribed or even extensive hypoechoic tumor localized in the mucosa (m type) or in the submucosa (sm type), with or without evidence of lymph node involvement. In contrast to the definition of early esophageal carcinoma, adjacent lymph node involvement in an early gastric carcinoma may be present. Overstaging may occur in the presence of peritumoral inflammation which cannot be distinguished from carcinomatous infiltration on ultrasound.[7,8]

T2 carcinoma appears as a hypoechoic tumor penetrating the adjacent muscularis propria or subserosal layer. Understaging in imaging may occur in the presence of microscopic infiltration (microinvasion) into the subserosal layer with intact continuity of the muscularis propria. Overstaging may occur in the case of deep infiltration of carcinoma into the muscularis propria without penetration into the serosal layer.

The diagnosis of T3 carcinoma may be difficult when the serosal layer cannot be imaged. In the presence of ascites, however, infiltration into the subserosal layer can be clearly imaged. In general, distinction between the subserosal and serosal layers with EUS is not possible. Moreover, the stomach is not entirely covered with peritoneum. Therefore, distinction between a T2 cancer and a T3 carcinoma is generally very difficult. I personally believe that distinction between minimal transmural tumor just beyond the muscularis propria, with extension less than 1 cm, and a deep transmural carcinoma with penetration more than 1 cm should be made based on the depth of infiltration in a way similar to those of ampullary carcinoma.

T4 carcinoma is often identified as deep penetration into the adjacent organs such as liver, pancreas, spleen, or structures such as major blood vessels, splenic artery, superior mesenteric artery, descending aorta, inferior vena cava, or portal vein (hepatoduodenal ligament). Some surgeons believe that in cases of proximal gastric cancer, particularly cardia carcinoma, involvement of the left gastric artery (lga) or the crus of diaphragm should be considered to be nonresectable.

In the assessment of regional lymph nodes, accurate measurement of the distance between the edge of the tumor and lymph nodes is obligatory. Lymph nodes less than 3 cm from the edge of tumor are defined as N1 and those more than 3 cm as N2. The most characteristic finding for metastasis is direct penetration of the carcinoma into adjacent lymph nodes.

In our series, the overall accuracy of EUS in diagnosing regional lymph nodes was 71%; sensitivity was 86% and specificity 47%. The low specificity results from false-positive diagnoses. The positive predictive value was 81% and negative predictive value 67%.[7] The accuracy of EUS in staging regional lymph nodes of gastric carcinoma is lower than that with esophageal carcinoma.[8] This is probably due to the more difficult route in identifying regional lymph nodes along with stomach and adjacent major blood vessels as compared to periesophageal lymph nodes. In the evaluation of distant metastases, EUS is less accurate because of the limited penetration depth of ultrasound. The right lobe of the liver cannot be assessed accurately and transcutaneous ultrasound is, therefore, always recommended in assessing distant metastasis. Peritoneal metastases or even direct penetration of tumor into the peritoneum may be diagnosed in the presence of ascites. This is done by imaging the bursa omentalis, although the major omentum may also be imaged. This permits visualization of solitary or diffuse peritoneal dissemination.

Feature of Gastric Linitis

Linitis plastica is a diffuse submucosal infiltrating gastric carcinoma, which often creates a very difficult differential diagnostic problem by endoscopy, barium swallow, and CT scan. The mucosa may be normal, diffusely thickened, or atrophic. Endoscopic biopsy may often be nondiagnostic because the tumor is buried deeply in the submucosa. Multiple biopsies taken from the same spot or biopsy with a giant biopsy forceps is often helpful in ascertaining the tissue diagnosis. EUS has a characteristic feature: the submucosa is obviously thickened two to four times as compared to those of normal gastric wall, diffuse hypoechoic infiltration is located in the submucosa, and the muscularis propria is often obviously thickened. The mucosal surface may show diffuse nodules.[19] Linitis can be found in the proximal or distal stomach or in the entire stomach. The first may extend its submucosal infiltration into the distal part of the esophagus, which should be accurately assessed prior to surgery. The latter may show distal extension into the pylorus and the duodenum. In female patients with gastric linitis metastatic involvement of the ovary may be found (Krukenberg tumor). A differential diagnosis between linitis and Ménétrier's disease or hypertrophic gastritis should be taken into consideration. The latter reveals a diffuse hypoechoic infiltration located at the mucosal level, whereas the submucosa is normal. In other words, the thickening of the gastric wall is primarily due to mucosal thickening. In linitis plastica, however, the thickening of the gastric wall is primarily due to the submucosal abnormality and secondarily due to the hypertrophy of the muscularis propria. With rapid advances of technology, EUS-guided cytology should be integrated in daily clinical practice in case of negative biopsy of diffuse gastric wall abnormalities. A positive tissue diagnosis is the final confirmation of malignancy.

Comments

The clinical stage (cTNM) is an expression of the anatomical extent of disease based on pretreatment clinical evaluation and microscopic examination of removed tissue. This can be assessed by EUS with biopsy and cytology. The pathological stages (pTNM classification) include the pretreatment clinical data plus additional evidence for pT and pN categories gleaned upon surgical resection and pathological examination of tissue.

In preoperative staging, EUS permits the most accurate assessment of the extent of tumor infiltration through the imaging of various sections of tumor. Moreover, regional lymph nodes can be imaged by maneuvering the echoprobe along the known anatomical site, usually adjacent to the corresponding blood vessels; classification on this basis has also recently been proposed by Japanese authors. EUS is also recommended before laser therapy for selecting appropriate patients and for documentation and follow-up after laser treatment. In our series, the accuracy of EUS in staging regional lymph node metastases in gastric carcinomas was lower than that in esophageal cancer. This may be explained by the more difficult route in identifying the perigastric lymph nodes compared with the periesophageal nodes. The most important criticism of gastric staging is the distinction between invasion into the subserosal layers and serosal layers. Anatomically, however, the stomach is not fully covered with a serosal layer such as the lesser curvature and the anterior side of the antrum. Probably, the depth of tumor infiltration into the subserosal layer should be used as a criterion in distinguishing a T2 from a T3 carcinoma comparable with those of ampullary cancer.

Case Report

In a 77-year-old man with cardiopulmonary insufficiency, endoscopy revealed a small malignant ulcer at the lesser curvature of the corpus of the stomach. Surgery was not recommended due to the patient's poor general condition. Initial EUS was performed before laser treatment revealed a hypoechoic tumor limited to the submucosa adjacent to the ulcer, consistent with an early gastric carcinoma. There was no evidence of regional lymph node involvement (T1N0). Follow-up EUS after laser therapy showed no evidence of local recurrence.

Case Report

A 66-year-old man was referred for endoscopy because of abdominal discomfort. Atrophic gastritis was found, without evidence of malignancy on endoscopy. During follow-up endoscopy because of progression of dysphagia, no malignant disorders were found. EUS revealed diffuse submucosal infiltration with penetration into the subserosa at the proximal stomach consistent with linitis plastica. The EUS findings were confirmed by the histology of the resected specimen.

Duodenum

Duodenal carcinomas are rare. Most carcinomas found by EUS are located in the descending part of the duodenum adjacent to the papilla of Vater. This intimate relationship to the papilla of Vater has also been described elsewhere.[20]

The investigation technique resembles that for gastric carcinomas. The tumor should first be identified endoscopically; thereafter the water-filled balloon method can be used. The most common exophytic tumor in the duodenum is villous adenoma. The site of villous adenomas varies, but the most common location is juxtapapillary. Detection of malignant degeneration in villous adenomas is generally difficult by endoscopy because multiple biopsies or piecemeal polypectomies may not always lead to the correct diagnosis. EUS may prove helpful in establishing the final diagnosis by guiding cytology or biopsy. Malignant degeneration appears on EUS as a hypoechoic pattern penetrating the submucosa and/or muscularis propria; this contrasts with the hyperechoic pattern of villous adenoma located in the mucosa.

The staging of duodenal carcinoma is comparable to that of gastric carcinoma. Carcinomas in the third portion of the duodenum may not be staged with EUS because the echoprobe cannot be positioned to the target of interest. (For practical reasons we do not discuss such rare carcinomas here but incorporate the subject in the section on the Ampulla of Vater, p 18.) This is particularly important for the surgeon because Whipple's resection is usually necessary to resect duodenal carcinoma due to the topographic relationship to the pancreas (retroperitoneal location). The long-term prognosis has been reported to be favorable, particularly in the early-stage carcinomas. The incidence of primary duodenal carcinoma is very low, approximately 1% of all cases of upper gastrointestinal carcinoma.

Case Report

In a 30-year-old man with polyposis coli associated with multiple gastric and duodenal polyps, a periampullary polyp was found with a diameter of 15 mm. Malignant tumor was not found on biopsy. EUS revealed intramucosal abnormalities without evidence of penetration into the submucosa or muscularis propria. Surgery was not recommended because the tissue diagnosis of malignancy was negative. During 2 years of follow-up, EUS showed no changes in size or in depth of tumor infiltration. Results of endoscopic biopsy were negative for carcinoma.

Case Report

A 38-year-old woman was referred for endoscopy because of abdominal discomfort and periodic epigastric pain. Laboratory investigation and transcutaneous abdominal ultrasound were nondiagnostic. Upper GI radiography revealed an extensive tumor mass with nodular appearance of the surface localized in the middle portion of the second part of the duodenum. Endoscopy revealed a mass protruding into the duodenal lumen. This mass was covered with a finely granular mucosa and was located proximal to the ampulla of Vater. Endosonography showed an extensive hypoechoic tumor located at the level of mucosa without penetration into the adjacent submucosal layer.[21] The muscularis propria was intact. No adjacent lymph node abnormality was found. The pancreatic duct, common bile duct, and pancreas were normal. The mass was diagnosed as a villous adenoma. After consultation with the surgeon a local tumor resection was preferred to a Whipple procedure because the tumor was limited to the mucosa. A longitudinal excision adjacent to the tumor margins was carried out and the tumor was locally resected. The ampulla of Vater was left intact. The histology of resected specimen revealed villous adenoma limited to the mucosa. Carcinomatous degeneration was not found and the tumor resection was radical. Eight days after surgery the patient was discharged.

The case demonstrates the crucial role of EUS in designing the strategy of treatment on the basis of the depth of abnormalities, whereas other imaging modalities fail.

Pancreas

Technique

The transgastric approach allows clear imaging of the body and tail of the pancreas as a result of the topographic anatomical relationship between the stomach and the pancreas. Examination of the entire head of the pancreas usually requires both transduodenal and transgastric approaches. The configuration of the stomach plays a crucial role for imaging of the pancreas.[5] A long, extended stomach provides clear visualization of the entire pancreas. In the case of a partially resected stomach, particularly by Billroth II operation imaging of the body and tail of the pancreas is still possible, but the periampullary region and the head of the pancreas cannot be imaged. On the other hand, adequate imaging of the entire pancreas may be possible in a stomach having undergone a Billroth I operation. Patients who had a total gastrectomy should not undergo EUS because the pancreas cannot be visualized ultrasonographically. For accurate imaging of the pancreas exact knowledge of the topographic anatomy is necessary. Moreover, extensive experience with transcutaneous abdominal ultrasound is required.

The most important landmark for the transgastric approach is the splenic vein, dorsal to the body and tail of the pancreas. The entire splenic vein can be followed from the splenoportal confluence to the splenic hilum. The left renal vein can be identified as a parallel vein immediately dorsal to the splenic vein, where it enters the left kidney. The splenic artery is ventral to the splenic vein, adjacent to the posterior wall of the stomach. The pancreatic duct is visualized approximately 1 cm ventral to the splenic vein.

By transduodenal approach, the head of the pancreas is visualized between the duodenal wall and the splenic vein or the superior mesenteric vein. The uncinate process is visualized adjacent to the mesenteric vessels and the aorta. The uncinate process should be placed dorsally (at the bottom of the screen) to achieve cross-sectional images analogous to those of CT. Careful examination of the entire uncinate region is recommended to detect mesenteric involvement, which is inevitably nonresectable at surgery. The gastroduodenal artery may occasionally be identified as a blood vessel originating from the mesenteric artery or hepatic artery.

Interpretation

The value of EUS lies principally in the comparison of its images to those of ERCP. Detailed knowledge of the anatomy of the pancreas is mandatory, particularly in identifying retroperitoneal blood vessels. The interpretation of pancreatic carcinomas follows the lines of that of transcutaneous ultrasonography. Classifying ductular abnormalities requires the incorporation of criteria used for the interpretation of ERCP.

Pancreatic carcinoma appears as a hypoechoic tumor usually obstructing the main Wirsung's duct, associated with a post-stenotic ductular dilation of the pancreatic duct and common bile duct. Intraductular tumors originating from the wall of the pancreatic duct are occasionally found. The intraductal polypoid pattern may represent proliferation of epithelium of the pancreatic duct and/or the carcinoma itself. Carcinoma in the uncinate process may cause ductular obstruction of the side branches without involvement of the main pancreatic duct. This may not always be seen on ERCP. Invasive neoplasms growing into the adjacent pancreatic parenchyma can be identified as a hypoechoic pattern adjacent to the dilated duct.

Criteria for assessing lymph node metastasis are described in previous chapters.

Definition

T: Primary tumor
T1: Hypoechoic tumor limited to the pancreas
    T1a: Tumor 2 cm or less in greatest dimension
    T1b: Tumor more than 2 cm in greatest dimension
T2: Tumor extending directly to duodenum, bile duct, or peripancreatic tissue
T3: Tumor extending directly to stomach, spleen, colon, or adjacent large vessels
    Tx: Primary tumor cannot be assessed.

N: Regional lymph nodes
N0: No regional lymph node metastasis
N1: Regional lymph node metastasis
    Nx: Regional lymph nodes cannot be assessed.

M: Distant metastasis
M0: No distant metastasis
M1: Distant metastasis: hepatic metastasis or peritoneal dissemination
    Mx: Distant metastasis cannot be assessed.

Stage grouping
Stage I: T1 N0 M0, T2 N0 M0
Stage II: T3 N0 M0
Stage III: Any T, N1 M0
Stage IV: Any T, any N M1

The pancreatic carcinoma adjacent to the abnormal pancreatic duct and common bile duct causes the so-called double-duct lesion seen by ERCP. Although the extent of tumor cannot be assessed by ERCP, it can be imaged by EUS. The tumor appears more hypoechoic than the surrounding tissue adjacent to the dilated common bile duct and pancreatic duct. In the case of carcinoma of the body and/or tail of the pancreas, obstruction of the common bile duct is rare except when an extensive tumor mass is found. The new TNM classification should be used for staging carcinomas only of the head of the pancreas (personal communication, P. Hermanek, Dept. of Surgery, University Hospital, Erlangen, Germany). Therefore, the bile duct and duodenum are used as demarcation points for T2 carcinoma. In our series, early intraductal carcinoma was found in the junction between the head and body of the pancreas more frequently than in the pancreatic head. Thus, no symptoms of jaundice or pruritus were present and abdominal discomfort and back pain were the initial symptoms. A small carcinoma located in the uncinate process, even one with a diameter of 2 cm, may show invasion into the adjacent blood vessels due to its close topographic anatomical relationship. Radical removal of carcinoma may be impossible.

Infiltration into the stomach is classified as a T3 carcinoma. This is the essential criterion of infiltration by carcinomas located in the head of the pancreas as a result of extensive growth. Carcinoma penetrating adjacent major blood vessels, particularly the splenoportal confluence, superior mesenteric vein or artery, splenic vein, or portal vein is also classified as T3. These blood vessels can be imaged clearly because of the real-time technique and the ability to assess various sections. Obstruction of the splenic vein due to extensive carcinoma, usually located in the body or tail of the pancreas, may cause portal hypertension with fundal varices of the stomach (segmental portal hypertension).[22] Occasionally ascites is found. This is an obvious contraindication for surgical resection.[23] Gastric varices are imaged as a hypoechoic ductular-like pattern in the submucosa usually associated with collateral veins. Compression by the tumor may be difficult to distinguish from carcinomatous infiltration based solely on the echo pattern. In the near future, the addition of a Doppler probe to EUS will probably enhance its accuracy in the assessment of vascular involvement. This is already widely used in the fields of echocardiography and transcutaneous abdominal ultrasound. The status of carcinomatous infiltration into the splenoportal confluence is essential for the further planning of surgical therapy. Vascular involvement appears as an irregularity in the vascular wall with partial or total obstruction of the lumen. This abnormality can be assessed by comparing the abnormal and normal vascular structures. The most important site of tumor invasion is the ipsilateral side of splenoportal confluence usually adjacent to or seldom contralateral to the duodenal lumen. For assessment or portal invasion, the dilated common bile duct can be used as a landmark.

Early pancreatic carcinoma is defined as T1 carcinoma (diameter under 2 cm) when there is no evidence of lymph node involvement. Such small carcinomas, however, are rare and may sometimes be found during the evaluation of patients with abdominal discomfort or back pain suspected of having pancreatic disease. The term "early cancer" as referred to for pancreatic cancer is controversial because of the high incidence of regional lymph node metastasis. In patients with obstructive jaundice, the carcinoma is usually found in advanced stages. Carcinoma in the uncinate process occasionally shows deep penetration into a mesocolon. This, however, may not be seen on EUS because of the difficulty in identifying the mesocolon except when ascites is present. This kind of fluid collection may stretch the mesocolon and make the imaging of its tumor invasion possible.

The uncinate process is located between the mesenteric vessels and the aorta. Careful examination of the uncinate process using the aorta and mesenteric vessels as landmarks is thus recommended. On ERCP, obstruction with corresponding ductal dilation of the side branches of the uncinate process may be found, occasionally with normal appearance of the main Wirsung's duct. Obstruction of the intrapancreatic common bile duct, however, may be present.

In our clinical experience, the incidence of lymph node involvement in T1 carcinoma is approximately 40–50%, which has also been reported elsewhere.[9,22,24] The incidence of lymph node metastasis increases with the progression of tumor infiltration. This may explain the poor prognosis of the disease.

The accuracy of EUS in the assessment of regional lymph nodes is comparable to that of esophagogastric carcinoma, but the assessment of distant metastasis with EUS is less accurate for the reasons mentioned in previous sections. Additional transcutaneous abdominal ultrasound with fine-needle aspiration cytology or biopsy of the liver is a valuable adjunct to EUS. In Europe, CT and magnetic resonance imaging for staging gastrointestinal tumors is less preferred than transcutaneous abdominal ultrasound, presumably because of the cost-benefit ratio, but in the United States and Canada, CT has become a standard procedure for staging pancreatic cancer. Carcinomas staged with these imaging techniques, however, are usually already in advanced stages.

Early stages of carcinoma should be treated surgically, whenever possible because of the highly malignant nature of the disease. Advanced stages, on the other hand, should be treated palliatively although the surgical approach may be considered after exact preoperative staging and biliary decompression with endoscopic drainage. In the near future, EUS-guided cytological puncture will be performed on lymph nodes suspected of malignancy. If the result is positive, surgical resection should be performed only in selected patients, for example, those of young age or without evidence of invasion into adjacent tissue.

Feature of Mucin-Producing Pancreatic Carcinoma

Mucin-producing pancreatic carcinoma has a relatively specific feature during ERCP and EUS. During ERCP an extremely dilated pancreatic duct with some intraductal filling defects can be observed. Mucin secretion through the ampulla may be seen, which represents the presence of high pressure within the pancreatic duct due to its excessive mucin production. On EUS the pancreatic duct is visualized as an extensive dilated duct with some protein-like plaque. The ductal mucosa may be flat or polypoid (Figure 47). Side branches may also be dilated. The size of the pancreatic duct may be larger than those of the splenic vein. Distinction between a mucin-producing pancreatic carcinoma and a cystadenoma or a cystadenocarcinoma is difficult. The latter may show a pattern similar in regards to the pancreatic duct in size, tortuosity of the duct, and ductal abnormality as compared with that of mucin-producing pancreatic carcinoma. Cystic dilation of side branches can often be found. The content of the pancreatic juice is more fluid-like rather than mucoid, which resembles a lesser degree of debris compared to that of mucin-producing tumor. The presence of extremely dilated pancreatic duct may simulate the diagnosis of pancreatic pseudocyst. Use of real-time ultrasound and careful examination of the extent of the pancreatic duct are often helpful in making a correct diagnosis. A dilated ductal structure with its tortuosity usually with some microcystic dilation of the side branches is strongly suggestive of cystadenoma or cystadenocarcinoma. An isolated or multiple extraductal cystic lesion with or without communication with the pancreatic duct is indicative of a pancreatic pseudocyst. The differential diagnosis between a cystadenoma and a cystadenocarcinoma is much more difficult or often impossible based solely on EUS pattern. Cholangioscopy with biopsy may become very helpful in ascertaining the final diagnosis. Determination of the value of EUS-guided fine needle aspiration must await further studies. In case of extremely dilated pancreatic duct, transductal EUS may be performed during ERCP or cholangioscopy.

Comments

Pancreatic carcinoma is a highly malignant disease with poor long-term prognosis. The incidence of lymph node metastasis even in early-stage carcinoma is high (30–40%). In the near future, tissue diagnosis by EUS-guided cytology of lymph nodes will play an important role in planning the strategy of treatment. Many surgeons consider surgery not to be indicated in the case of positive cytology for liver metastasis. The clinical value of EUS in the detection of early pancreatic carcinomas is still unknown because only few cases have been reported.[9,10] At present, EUS does not appear to be an appropriate diagnostic screening modality because of the invasive nature of the procedure and the unfavorable cost–benefit ratio. Rosch et al. reported that EUS was superior to angiography, CT, and abdominal ultrasonography (US) (EUS 95%, angiography 85%, CT 75%, and US 55%).[25] Snady et al. reported that EUS was significantly more accurate than combined CT and ERCP with an accuracy of 75% and 38%, respectively.[26] Recently, we reported the use of EUS-guided cytology in diagnosing and staging pancreatic cancer invading the gastric wall, which could not be diagnosed by endoscopy and CT.[27] In this reported series segmental portal hypertension due to tumor invasion was stressed to be an unresectable criterion and surgery should not be attempted.

Case Report

A 70-year-old man was referred because of abdominal discomfort and back pain. Cholestasis was not found, gastroscopy showed no abnormality, and ERCP revealed complete obstruction of the main pancreatic duct—strongly suspect for extensive carcinoma. EUS imaged a polypoid intraductal tumor with some penetration into the adjacent pancreatic parenchyma. The diameter of the tumor was approximately 20 mm. No evidence of lymph node involvement was found (Figure 43). Other imaging modalities (transcutaneous ultrasound, CT, angiography) failed to identify the tumor. After consultation with the surgeon distal pancreatectomy was performed because of the chance of curative resection. The histology of resected specimen confirmed the diagnosis of EUS as T1 N0. During 3-year clinical follow-up the patient was doing well and no recurrent tumor was found.

Thus, in the case of small pancreatic carcinoma EUS can be expected to become the trend in the near future for staging the anatomical extent of carcinoma and for detecting regional lymph node metastasis.

Ampulla of Vater

Carcinomas of the ampulla of Vater are reported to have a more favorable prognosis than pancreatic carcinomas. The clinical symptoms are similar to those of pancreatic cancer, but the early onset of those symptoms, such as jaundice, results in a relatively high proportion of tumors being diagnosed with early stage of disease. Distinction between ampullary carcinomas and pancreatic cancers is important because of the different long-term prognosis and is necessary in planning the strategy of treatment. Histologically, ampullary carcinomas can resemble duodenal tumors or distal bile duct cancers. Since ampullary carcinomas resemble specifically localized duodenal adenocarcinoma, TNM classification of ampullary carcinoma is particularly meaningful.

Technique

The technique is similar to that for examination of the head of the pancreas. The papilla should be found endoscopically, after which the echoprobe is placed adjacent to the target lesion. The instrument should be stretched along the lesser curvature. The characteristic anatomical architecture of the papilla of Vater is a nodular or polypoid nodular ampulla, usually containing the common channel with a bifurcation into the corresponding pancreatic duct and common bile duct. Anatomical variants of the ampulla of Vater regarding the configuration of the common channel, however, should be taken into consideration. The most important landmarks in the staging of a carcinoma are the muscularis of the papilla and the penetration into the common bile duct or the adjacent pancreas or duodenum. Lymph nodes along the common bile duct and the portal vein and in the pancreatic head should be examined carefully. Moreover, lymph nodes at the splenic hilum should be identified in order to stage the presence or absence of distant metastasis.

Definition

T: Primary tumor
T1:   Tumor limited to ampulla of Vater
T2:   Tumor invading duodenal wall
T3:   Tumor invading 2 cm or less into pancreas
T4:   Tumor invading more than 2 cm into pancreas or other adjacent organs
       Tx: Primary tumor cannot be assessed.

N: Regional lymph nodes
N0:   No regional lymph node metastasis
N1:   Regional lymph node metastasis
       Nx: Regional lymph nodes not assessable

M: Distant metastasis
M0:   No distant metastasis
M1:   Distant metastasis: hepatic metastasis, peritoneal dissemination, or lymph node metastasis along the splenic vein or at the splenic hilum
       Mx: Distant metastasis not assessable

Stage grouping
Stage I: T1 N0 M0
Stage II: T2 N0 M0, T3 N0 M0
Stage III: T1 N1 M0, T2 N1 M0, T3 N1 M0
Stage IV: T4, any N M0, any T, any N M1

EUS permits accurate evaluation of the depth of tumorous infiltration in ampullary carcinoma because of its ability to image the anatomical structure of the ampulla of Vater as well as the common bile duct and the pancreatic duct. EUS can also be used to image ductal abnormalities found by ERCP. Ductal dilation is usually caused by tumor infiltration but may also be due to compression by involved or enlarged lymph nodes. Dilation of bile duct can be imaged easily before insertion of a biliary stent for decompression. In cases following biliary stenting, the extent of tumor involvement can be imaged accurately using the stent as a landmark. The stent appears within the tumor mass as two hyperechoic (white) lines, representing the partial reflection of the ultrasound beam at the surface of the stent.

T1 carcinoma appears as a hypoechoic pattern in the mucosa, sphincter muscle, or submucosal layer of the ampulla of Vater. There must be no evidence of penetration into the muscularis propria of the adjacent duodenal wall.

T2 carcinoma is defined as a hypoechoic tumor invading the duodenal wall. This indicates that the muscularis propria of the duodenum has been penetrated.

T3 and T4 carcinomas are defined by the depth of infiltration into the pancreatic parenchyma; a depth of 2 cm characterizes T3 carcinoma and one of more than 2 cm T4 carcinoma. In such cases, ampullary carcinoma cannot be distinguished from pancreatic cancer solely on the basis of echo pattern and anatomical extent; even with histology one may not always be able to determine the final diagnosis.

The most important advantage of this technique is its ability to distinguish ampullary carcinoma from pancreatic cancer, particularly in the early stages of disease. This is important in selecting appropriate patients for the Whipple type of pancreatic resection. Moreover, cytological puncture may further enhance the diagnostic value of EUS in cases of questionable diagnosis.

Lymph nodes at the splenic hilum should be examined carefully to identify distant metastasis. The reason for classifying involvement of these lymph nodes as metastatic disease lies in their distance from the primary site of carcinomas.

In our series involving 24 cases with ampullary carcinoma, the accuracy of EUS in assessing T1 tumors was 67%, T2 tumors 92%, T3 tumors 87%, and T4 tumors 100%. The overall accuracy rate was 87%. In diagnosing benign regional lymph nodes in ampullary carcinomas the accuracy was only 54%. For diagnosing metastatic lymph nodes, however, the accuracy was 80%. The prevalence of lymph node metastases in T1 ampullary carcinoma was 0%. Similar to our previous results in staging gastroesophageal and pancreatic cancers, EUS is not accurate in staging distant metastases.

The 5-year survival rate correlates with the stage of the stage of carcinoma. Early stage carcinomas have a much better prognosis than that of advanced cancers. According to the pathologic TNM classification of resected specimen (pTNM), survival of stage I tumors was 100%.[23] Interestingly, local tumor resection has been reported to result in better 5-year survival rates than Whipple resection.[25] Recently, minimally invasive surgery has been propagated for the treatment of superficially limited gastroesophageal tumors. This might be attempted for an intra-mucosal ambullary carcinoma particularly in high risk patients such as elderly or cardiopulmonally illea patients.

Comments

Ampullary carcinoma has become clinically important as a result of its similarity to pancreatic cancer in terms of symptoms, initial endoscopic treatment, and surgical approach but the difference between the two in terms of the strategy of further treatment should be stressed. In general, Whipple's resection should be preferred over endoscopic palliation except in very advanced stages of the disease. The use of EUS to distinguish between early- and advanced-stage carcinomas is one of the most important topics in preoperative staging. Occasionally, differentiation be-tween mucosal and submucosal ampullary carcinoma is possible. The former may have a more favorable long-term prognosis, and a local resection without Whip-ple's procedure may be considered. The philosophy of such treatment is based on that of early gastric cancer. The presence of lymph node involvement, however, should be ruled out with EUS prior to the therapy.

Case Report

A 50-year-old man was referred for transcutaneous abdominal ultrasound to screen for gallstone disease because of recurrent abdominal discomfort at the upper right quadrant. No itching or jaundice was present. Dilation of bile ducts was found without evidence of tumor mass in the pancreas or liver metastases. The gallbladder was normal. ERCP was unsuccessful due to a pedunculated ampullary tumor that was confirmed to be carcinoma on biopsy. EUS revealed a pedunculated polyp with a small hypoechoic tumor limited to the mucosa without evidence of penetration into the stalk (Figure 37). There was no evidence of lymph node metastases. Local tumor resection without Whipple's procedure was recommended and performed. The histology of the resected specimen confirmed the EUS finding compatible with a T1 carcinoma. Follow-up EUS after 3 months revealed no evidence of tumor or lymph node involvement. Further follow-up after a period of 18 months was performed. EUS and endoscopic biopsy did not show evidence of tumor recurrence. This case clearly demonstrates the uniqueness of EUS.[28]

Distal Extrahepatic Bile Duct

Cholangiocarcinomas are reported to grow slowly and seldom to entail distant metastases, which should result in a more favorable long-term prognosis than is the case with pancreatic carcinomas. Recent studies, however, show a relatively poor long-term prognosis for the disease. The increasing frequency of cholangio-carcinomas currently being found preoperatively reflects improvements in diagnostic imaging modalities.

Technique

The investigation technique is similar to the previously described method for examination of the head of the pancreas and the ampulla of Vater. Approached trans-duodenally, the most important landmarks are the portal vein, splenic vein, superior mesenteric vein, and head of the pancreas. The dilated common bile duct can be visualized directly adjacent to the duodenal wall and ventral to the portal vein. By slow withdrawal of the instrument, the extrahepatic duct can be followed to the liver hilum. The cystic duct and the gallbladder can usually be recognized relative to the duodenal bulb and/or the antrum of the stomach. The portal vein, splenic vein, superior mesenteric vein, and particularly the confluence of these veins should be examined carefully for accurate assessment in staging the carcinoma.

Definition

T: Primary tumor
T1:   Tumor invading mucosa or muscle layer
    T1a: Tumor invading mucosa
    T1b: Tumor invading muscle layer
T2:   Tumor invading perimuscular connective tissue
T3:   Tumor invading adjacent structures: liver, pancreas, duodenum, gallbladder, colon, or stomach

N: Regional lymph nodes
N0:   No regional lymph node metastasis
N1:   Regional lymph node metastasis
    N1a: Lymph node along the common bile duct and cystic duct and in the hilum of the liver
    N1b: Periduodenal, periportal, adjacent to the celiac trunk and mesenteric blood vessels

M: Distant metastasis
M0:   No distant metastasis
M1:   Distant metastasis: peritoneal dissemination, hepatic metastasis, or perigastric lymph nodes

Stage grouping
Stage I: T1 N0 M0
Stage II: T2 N0 M0, T3 N0 M0
Stage III: T1 N1 M0, T2 N1 M0, T3 N1 M0
Stage IV: T4 any N M0, any T any N M1

The most characteristic finding of distal bile duct carcinoma is an intramural and/or transmural hypoechoic pattern in the common bile duct, with prestenotic dilation of the bile duct but no evidence of penetration into the adjacent pancreatic tissue or duct. In the case of involvement of the adjacent pancreatic duct, distinction between a distal common bile duct carcinoma and a pancreatic cancer may become difficult or even impossible. When ampullary carcinoma with infiltration into the adjacent common bile duct results in prestenotic dilation, there may be some difficulty to distinguish it from an extrahepatic common bile duct carcinoma. One occasionally finds villous adenomas of the common bile duct (T0), which may result in findings upon ERCP and EUS that are similar to those in carcinomas. In the future, choledochoscopy with biopsy can be expected to provide help in establishing the final diagnosis. Histologic assessment and cytology performed during ERCP may not always determine the final diagnosis.

T1 carcinoma of the common bile duct appears as a hypoechoic intraductal tumor without evidence of penetration into the adjacent muscularis propria of the bile duct associated with dilation of the corresponding bile duct. Adjacent lymph nodes may already be involved by metastatic tissue. Clinical symptoms of T1 carcinoma, such as jaundice, are extremely rare, probably because of incomplete biliary obstruction.

T2 carcinoma appears as a hypoechoic tumor with transmural infiltration but without evidence of infiltration into adjacent structures. Cholangiocarcinoma associated with peritumoral pancreatitis often cannot be distinguished from pancreatic cancer solely on the basis of the echo pattern. In such cases, a double-duct lesion can be imaged on ultrasound, which may simulate the presence of pancreatic cancer or penetration of bile duct carcinoma into the pancreas (overstaging).

T3 carcinoma appears as a hypoechoic tumor penetrating into the adjacent portal vein and/or pancreas and is usually associated with involvement of adjacent lymph nodes.

In our series of 33 cases with bile duct carcinoma that underwent surgery for Whipple resection, the accuracy of EUS for T1 cancers was 100% (n = 2), in T2 cancers 80%, and in T3 cancers 81.8%. The overall accuracy was 82.8%.[11] In contrast to local tumor resection for superficial ampullary cancers, T1 common bile duct tumors require a Whipple resection because of their difficult anatomical location and the more aggressive nature of the disease. In the near future cholangioscopy may become essential in achieving a tissue diagnosis particularly in distinguishing adenomas from carcinomas in the bile duct. Combination of transpapillary EUS using a miniature catheter echoprobe and cholangioscopy will hopefully become the trend in the future. At present, however, even adenomyomatosis of the common bile duct still requires Whipple resection because of the difficulty in achieving the final diagnosis prior to surgery.

Comments

Our clinical experience shows EUS to be helpful in detecting early-stage disease. Intraductal polypoid tumors limited to the wall of the common bile duct are consistent with a T1 carcinoma, a villous adenoma or an adenomyomatosis. The final diagnosis remains the tissue diagnosis by biopsy or a positive final needle aspiration for malignancy. Transmural tumors with direct extension into the pericholedochal connective tissue are strongly suspicious of malignancy. Lymph nodes directly adjacent to the tumor are occasionally also found. Advanced stages can be diagnosed by the presence of penetration into adjacent pancreas, duodenum, and the gallbladder. The most important advantage of this technique is its ability to detect the early stage of carcinoma and nonresectable carcinomas. Tumor invasion into the major blood vessels indicates nonresectability of lesions. Disadvantages include the limited penetration depth of ultrasound and the difficulty in maneuvering the transducer into the duodenum to produce adequate cross-sectional ultrasound images. Moreover, extensive training in endoscopy and transcutaneous ultrasound is necessary for adequate interpretation of ultrasound images.

Case Report

A 68-year-old man was referred for ERCP because of dilation of extrahepatic duct found by abdominal ultrasound. ERCP revealed some polypoid filling defects in the distal common bile duct and prominent papilla of Vater. The biopsy was positive for carcinoma. EUS revealed longstanding polypoid intraductal tumor in the common hepatic duct. No evidence of lymph node metastases was found. The patient underwent a Whipple's resection because a local tumor resection alone was not possible due to its anatomical location. Histology confirmed the EUS findings consistent with T1 carcinoma.

Proximal Extrahepatic Bile Duct

Proximal bile duct carcinomas are often found adjacent to the bifurcation of hepatic ducts (the so-called Klatskin tumor). Obstruction of the hepatic confluence in patients without previous biliary surgery is always suspect for malignancy. The most characteristic finding in Klatskin tumor on EUS is the hypoechoic intra- or transmural echo pattern surrounded by a hyperechoic fibrotic rim; this has been described macroscopically and histologically as a tumor surrounded by fibrotic tissue.[29,30] It may be difficult to assess the malignant nature of the tumor at surgery, even by histology of the removed specimen, because of its fibrotic character and difficult anatomical location. This type of obstruction is sometimes difficult to drain endoscopically. In cases of successful drainage, the biliary stent may clog, resulting in cholangitis. This makes endoscopic removal of the obstructed stent necessary and its replacement by a new large-channel endoprosthesis. Accurate preoperative staging is therefore of utmost importance, particularly determination of the anatomical extent of carcinoma, for selecting patients who might benefit from surgery or endoscopic drainage.

Technique

The technique of investigation corresponds to that previously described for distal common bile duct tumors. The most important landmarks are the portal vein and dilated hepatic bile ducts. A dilated common bile duct appears as an anechoic ductular structure between the gastrointestinal wall and the portal vein, situated ventral and parallel to the portal vein. The left hepatic duct system should be examined transgastrically. The topographic relationship between the stomach and the liver plays an important role in accurately visualizing the biliary system. An elongated stomach allows excellent transgastric visualization of the biliary system, whereas a partially resected stomach makes adequate examination difficult or even impossible. The examination should begin from the distal stomach along the lesser curvature, after which the echoprobe should be introduced into the duodenum. The distal common bile duct, the common hepatic duct, and the right hepatic duct can be imaged from the apex of the duodenum or at the proximal part of the second portion of duodenum. The gallbladder and the cystic duct should be visualized if possible. The relationship between the cystic duct and the common bile duct is variable and occasionally the cystic duct can be found in close proximity to the intrapancreatic portion of the common bile duct. Knowledge of the interpretation of ERCP images is essential for understanding the normal anatomy and pathology of the biliary tree. Ductal images comparable to ERCP radiographic pictures should be obtained for standardization of EUS images. The inserted endoprosthesis can readily be used as a landmark for identifying the primary tumor.

Interpretation

The same TNM classification used for distal duct carcinomas is used for proximal bile duct carcinoma. EUS criteria for assessing the primary tumor, regional lymph nodes, and distant metastasis are comparable to those described in the previous section.

T: Primary tumor
T1:   Hypoechoic intraductal tumor invading the mucosa or muscle layer
    T1a: Hypoechoic tumor invading the mucosa
    T1b: Hypoechoic tumor invading muscle layer (muscularis propria)
T2:   Hypoechoic tumor invading perimuscular hyperechoic tissue
T3:   Hypoechoic tumor invading adjacent structures: liver, gallbladder, adjacent portal vein, or hepatic artery
    Tx: Primary tumor cannot be assessed.

N: Regional lymph nodes
N0:   No regional lymph node metastasis
N1:   Regional lymph node metastasis
    N1a: Lymph nodes at the liver hilum adjacent to the cystic duct and/or common bile duct
    N1b: Periduodenal, adjacent to the celiac trunk and mesenteric blood vessels
    Nx: Regional lymph nodes cannot be assessed.

M: Distant metastasis
M0:   No distant metastasis
M1:   Distant metastasis: hepatic metastasis or peritoneal dissemination
    Mx: Distant metastasis cannot be assessed.

Stage Grouping

The definition of stage grouping corresponds to that of distal extrahepatic bile duct carcinoma.

Early stages of this disease are encountered extremely rarely because of the absence of jaundice and other symptoms; however, early carcinoma defined as T1 without evidence of lymph node involvement has been reported in a relatively large series in Japan.

T1 carcinoma appears as an intraductally growing pattern in the mucosa with or without penetration into the adjacent muscularis propria. Prestenotic dilation of the corresponding bile duct can be visualized. Dilation of both left and right systems is seen when the tumor is located at the bifurcation. Adjacent regional lymph nodes at the porta hepatis of T1 carcinoma are usually not involved.

T2 carcinoma appears as a hypoechoic tumor penetrating the wall but not adjacent structures. Carcinoma may spread along the bile duct lumen or may even metastatically involve the peripheral intrahepatic bile ducts (multifocal carcinomas). Adjacent regional lymph node metastases are usually found.

T3 carcinoma appears as a transmural hypoechoic tumor penetrating the adjacent liver parenchyma or portal vein. If the distal common hepatic duct adjacent to the cystic duct is involved, distinction between a bifurcation and a gallbladder carcinoma is not possible. Moreover, distal bile duct carcinoma may spread to the proximal or distal bile duct or into the gallbladder. In such cases, TNM staging may prove difficult. Courvoisier's sign is the most common finding in these clinically extensive cholangiocarcinomas, and they entail a very poor prognosis. Endoscopic stent placement is the preferred treatment whenever possible. In one of our

30 patients with histologically confirmed T3 Klatskin tumor, direct intraductal tumor spreading through the cystic duct into the wall of the gallbladder was found, contrasting with a transmural tumor spreading through the connective tissue into the gallbladder.[11] The latter has a similar feature of gallbladder carcinoma found during explorative surgery or histologically by examination of resected specimen.

Comments

The recently reported increase in the number of Klatskin tumors is presumably due to the improvement in diagnostic modalities. Such carcinomas usually have a relatively good long-term prognosis when decompression of the obstructed biliary system is successfully performed. Deaths result from cholangitis or liver failure rather than from the primary disease. ERCP and percutaneous transhepatic cholangiography (PTC) are accurate techniques for assessing abnormalities in the ductular system, but they do not permit imaging of the anatomical extent of disease. CT and transcutaneous ultrasound are accurate for visualizing ductular dilation but not the primary site of tumor, presumably because of the similar density of echo pattern in the primary lesion and the surrounding tissue. Therefore, EUS is the most valuable imaging technique to assess both ductal abnormalities and the anatomical extent of disease. However, malignant diseases such as metastases, non-Hodgkin's lymphoma, and hepatoma and benign disorders such as fibrosis and Mirizzi's syndrome may show similar ductular abnormalities and tumoral echo patterns comparable to those of bifurcation carcinomas of the hepatic duct. Examination of tissue is necessary for the final diagnosis. The definition of T3 carcinoma as tumor invasion into the gallbladder requires further classification. In my opinion, intraductal tumor spreading along the cystic duct into the gallbladder should be defined as T2 carcinoma, and transmural tumor spreading through the connective tissue into the gallbladder as T3 carcinoma spreading into the common hepatic duct and cystic duct. This hypothesis, however, needs further clarification through long-term studies with a large number of patients. We have found a high incidence of Klatskin tumor among relatively young patients in our series, which has been published elsewhere.[30]

In our series of 43 cases that underwent surgery no T1 Klatskin tumor was found; probably, such superficial cancers do not cause biliary obstruction. Obstructive jaundice is almost always associated with an advanced stage carcinoma. The accuracy of EUS in T2 and T3 cancers was 70% and 90%, respectively.[11] The difficulty was in distinguishing tumor compression from tumor invasion.[11] We have found an interesting observation regarding the prevalence of lymph node metastasis. In common bile duct cancer, the incidence increased with the progression of the depth of tumor invasion. In Klatskin tumor, however, such correlation was not found. In biopsy-negative proximal bile duct obstruction, malignancy other than carcinoma such as non-Hodgkin's lymphoma, leiomyosarcoma, or benign diseases such as sclerosing cholangitis or purulent cholangitis with formation of microabscesses should be taken into consideration.

Case Report

A 30-year-old man was referred for surgery because of obstruction in the proximal extrahepatic duct. Preoperative EUS revealed multiple, intraductal spreading bile duct carcinomas, located principally in the bifurcation of bile ducts. No lymph node involvement was found. The patient underwent tumor resection with extended liver resection. The EUS findings were confirmed. Although the tumors were mainly intraductal, the patient died from diffuse tumor recurrence due to multifocal spread.

Gallbladder

Technique

It is sometimes not possible to visualize the gallbladder transgastrically or transduo-denally because of topographic anatomical variations between the gallbladder and gastroduodenal tract and the limited depth of ultrasound. The gallbladder adjacent to the stomach and duodenum can readily be found by maneuvering the echoprobe into the duodenum or by withdrawing the instrument along the lesser curvature of the stomach. The normal gallbladder appears as an anechoic cavity with smooth thin wall. The first hyperechoic structure corresponds to the interface between the bile and the mucosa and the second (hypoechoic) structure to the muscularis of the gallbladder. The third hyperechoic structure corresponds to the periconnective tissue and the interface echos. Interface echos, however, should be taken into consideration for the interpretation; their thickness is related to the axial resolution of the transducer.

Interpretation

Carcinoma of the gallbladder appears as a small nodular or polypoid tumor with continuity to the wall of the gallbladder. Advanced carcinoma is visualized as an extensive, deeply penetrating hypoechoic mass usually invading the adjacent duodenal wall and the liver hilum.

T: Primary tumor
T1:   Small hypoechoic nodular or polypoid tumor originating from the wall of the gallbladder, without evidence of penetration into the muscularis propria
T2:   Hypoechoic tumor penetrating the adjacent muscle layer
T3:   Hypoechoic tumor deeply penetrating the adjacent structures such as duodenum, liver, or major blood vessels
Tx: Primary tumor cannot be assessed.

N: Regional lymph nodes
N0:   No regional lymph node metastasis
N1:   Regional lymph node metastasis
Nx: Regional lymph nodes cannot be assessed.

M: Distant metastasis
M0:   No distant metastasis
M1:   Distant metastasis: hepatic metastasis or peritoneal dissemination
Mx: Distant metastasis cannot be assessed.

Stage grouping
Stage I: T1 N0 M0
Stage II: T2 N0 M0
Stage III: T1 N1 M0, T2 N1 M0, T3 N1 M0
Stage IV: T4 any N M0, any T any N M1

The normal gallbladder wall appears as a hyperechoic pattern corresponding to the interface between the bile and the mucosa. The muscle layer produces a hypoechoic pattern surrounded by a hyperechoic structure.

T1 carcinoma appears as a small hypoechoic pattern with hypoechoic sur-rounding structures usually causing a small bulging lesion.

T2 carcinoma appears as a hypoechoic pattern penetrating the muscle layer and perimuscular connective tissue but not invading adjacent structures. Early stages of carcinoma may sometimes be detected in resected specimens of patients who have undergone surgery for gallstone disease.

T3 carcinoma appears as a transmural hypoechoic pattern penetrating deeply into the adjacent structures such as duodenum, liver, colonic segment, or major blood vessels. As mentioned above, tumor penetration into the proximal bile duct may simulate the presence of a Klatskin tumor. Moreover, Mirizzi's syndrome should be considered in the differential diagnosis of a mass obstructing the distal common hepatic bile duct without successful imaging of the gallbladder. In the case of deep penetration into the liver parenchyma, primary liver carcinoma should be taken into consideration. Cytology guided by transcutaneous ultrasound or histology may be helpful in determining the final diagnosis.

Case Report

A 68-year-old man with painless obstructive jaundice was referred for ERCP, CT, and EUS for evaluation. ERCP showed an obstruction in the middle part of common bile duct without filling the gallbladder and the proximal hepatic bile duct. The pancreatic duct showed a short segment consistent with ventral pancreas (pancreas divisum). The diagnosis of Klatskin tumor or gallbladder carcinoma was raised. CT showed a stone in the gallbladder without visualization of tumor in the gallbladder or at the bifurcation of hepatic bile ducts. EUS showed a hypoechoic tumor mass in the gallbladder adjacent to a hyperechoic gallstone. The tumor showed transmural infiltration with direct penetration into the adjacent duodenal submucosa. EUS-guided cytology using a modified sclerotherapy needle was positive for adenocarcinoma.[31] The EUS diagnosis was a T3 gallbladder carcinoma penetrating into the submucosa of the duodenum. Surgery was not recommended and endoscopic insertion of a biliary stent was the choice of treatment. This case illustrates clearly the uniqueness of EUS combined with aspiration cytology in case of duodenal submucosal invasion which cannot be diagnosed with other imaging modalities.[32]

PRIMARY TUMORS OF THE COLON AND RECTUM

Colorectal carcinoma has become one of the major causes of death in industrialized countries after lung and breast cancer. Those affected are generally over 40 years of age. In those younger than 35, colorectal cancer is often associated with polyposis coli or a family history of colorectal cancer.

The TNM classification for the colon and rectum applies only to carcinoma. Recently there has been a revision in the T categories and in the stage grouping of the TNM classification, permitting a direct translation to the Dukes' classification scheme. The N classification has been revised to include the location of involved lymph nodes. Both T and N changes were based on data from the Erlangen Tumor Registry. For reasons of clinical relevance the colon is divided into rectum (rectum and rectosigmoid junction) and proximal colonic segments (suprarectal colon). This distinction represents the technical aspect of EUS investigation: carcinomas of the former can be investigated with a nonoptic instrument (rigid or flexible equipment) whereas those of the latter should be examined with a fiberoptic echoendoscope (echoduodenoscope or echocolonoscope).

Instruments

An Aloka rigid or flexible instrument and an Olympus prototype fiberoptic echocolonoscope are available for colorectal EUS. The Aloka instrument has a rigid shaft

Table 2. Technical Features of Instruments for Examining Colorectal Carcinoma

	Nonoptic		Optic	
	Rigid	Flexible	Side-viewing	Forward-viewing
Length (cm)	12	65	120	130
Diameter (mm)	15	10	13	15
Frequency (MHz)	5	7.5	7.5	7.5
Penetration depth (cm)	22	10	10	10
Axial resolution (mm)	2	0.2	0.2	0.2

of 12 cm in length and a transducer at its tip, with a length of 5 cm and an outer diameter of 15 mm. The frequency of ultrasound in 5 MHz, penetration depth is approximately 22 cm, and axial resolution is 0.4 mm. The prototype Olympus echocolonoscope (XCF-UM2) has a small transducer attached just beyond the frontal-viewing optics. A biopsy channel adjacent to the transducer is available for biopsy or filling the colorectal lumen with water. I use the rigid Aloka ASU-59 and a flexible Aloka prototype to examine rectal carcinomas; for the sigmoid colon, I use the 10-MHz lateral-viewing echoendoscope. For examination of the more proximal colonic segments, I prefer the prototype echocoloscope (AXF-EUM2). To assess the sigmoid colon and the proximal colonic segments, I formerly used the lateral viewing echoendoscope but have recently tended increasingly to the forward-viewing echocoloscope since its forward view allows it to be more readily maneuvered endoscopically. For accurate ultrasound visualization, however, adequate filling of the colonic lumen with water is mandatory, as with the investigation of the stomach. This radial scanner has a sector only of approximately 330° because the location of the biopsy channel adjacent to the transducer hampers the transmission of ultrasound. The area under the biopsy channel cannot be seen due to the total reflection of the ultrasound beam. The newly available Olympus prototype echocoloscope may be attached with a water-filled balloon at the transducer that facilitates imaging of colorectal abnormalities. In the case of suspected penetration of rectal carcinoma into the posterior wall of the vagina, additional transvaginal EUS is helpful in determining the extent of tumor infiltration. Recently an Aloka sector vaginal echoprobe has become available. Table 2 summarizes the technical features of the instruments available.

Investigation Techniques

The technique for investigation of colorectal carcinoma resembles that of rectosigmoidoscopy, with patients lying in the left lateral decubital position following administration of a phosphate enema. Rectal digital examination is obligatory to assess the local anatomy of rectal cancer and to dilate the anal sphincter muscle prior to insertion of the instrument. The nonoptic instrument is inserted blindly as deeply as possible. Thereafter, the instrument should be withdrawn carefully until abnormalities are imaged. By filling the rectal lumen with water the polypoid or exophytic configuration of tumors can be clearly visualized. The method of investigation with the echoendoscope is similar to that for gastric carcinomas. For forward-viewing instruments the lumen must be filled with water because the tip of the instrument cannot be covered with a balloon, and a separate water channel for filling the balloon with water is not available. Whenever possible, the instrument should be passed beyond the lesion into the proximal colonic segments to visualize lymph node abnormalities and to determine the proximal tumor-free area. This is important to obtain accurate information in localizing the resection margins.

Rectum

The interpretation of the normal and pathological structures is based on the results of previous studies. The architecture of the colonic wall is similar to that of the gastric wall. In the rectum the continuous structure adjacent to the muscularis propria is subserosa; thus, there is no covering peritoneum. In the sigmoid colon the outer structure is the serosa.

Definition

T: Primary tumor
T1:   Tumor invading the mucosa or submucosa
T2:   Tumor invading muscularis propria
T3:   Tumor invading through muscularis propria into subserosa or into non-peritonealized pericolic or perirectal tissues
T4:   Tumor penetrating the visceral peritoneum or directly invading other organs or structures
    Tx: Primary tumor cannot be assessed.

N: Regional lymph nodes
N0:   No regional lymph node metastasis
N1:   Metastasis in one to three pericolic or perirectal lymph nodes
N2:   Metastasis in four or more pericolic or perirectal lymph nodes
N3:   Metastasis along the course of a named vascular trunk
    Nx: Regional lymph nodes cannot be assessed.

M: Distant metastasis
M0:   No distant metastasis
M1:   Distant metastasis: hepatic metastasis or peritoneal dissemination
    Mx: Distant metastasis cannot be assessed.

Stage grouping
Stage I: T1 N0 M0, T2 N0 M0
Stage II: T3 N0 M0, T4 N0 M0
Stage III: Any T N1 M0, any T N2 M0, any T N3 M0
Stage IV: Any T any N M1

The most common difficulty in endoscopy lies in distinguishing villous adenoma from villous adenoma with malignant degeneration (carcinoma). The malignancy is usually covered with nonmalignant villous tissue. Therefore, endoscopic biopsy may not always determine the diagnosis. By careful EUS examination of the tumorous mass, the malignancy can be imaged as a hypoechoic tumor penetrating the submucosa or muscularis propria (bowel wall).[33,34] In cases of intramucosal or intraepithelial malignancy, however, the EUS may not be able to distinguish the focal carcinoma from the surrounding villous tissue. Distinction between the villous adenomatous tissue and the muscularis mucosae is not possible on ultrasound, but penetration of malignant tissue into the adjacent submucosa, muscularis propria, or even the adjacent structures can readily be imaged. Malignant regional lymph nodes can also be visualized. We prefer to use an echocolonoscope to identify the target lesion endoscopically and thereafter to fill the lumen with water. EUS-guided biopsy or cytology can be used to establish the diagnosis histologically.

T1 carcinoma appears as a hypoechoic tumor in the mucosa or submucosa without penetration into the muscularis propria.

T2 carcinoma appears as a hypoechoic tumor penetrating into but not through the muscularis propria. Occasionally, the inner ring and outer longitudinal layer can be visualized separately with a hyperechoic fibrotic pattern appearing between the two muscle layers. In rectal carcinomas, overstaging may occur due to peritumoral inflammation, abscesses, or previous irradiation. Overstaging of T2 carcinoma with peritumoral inflammation or abscesses may thus be found more often in rectal than in suprarectal carcinoma.[12] In such cases, even high-frequency, high-resolution instruments may not be helpful because the muscle layer cannot be distinguished from the surrounding inflamed tissue. This hypothesis, however, should be confirmed by clinical studies.

T3 carcinoma appears as a hypoechoic tumor penetrating the subserosal layer but not adjacent structures. The peritoneal layer can be identified only by the presence of ascites.

T4 carcinoma appears as a hypoechoic tumor penetrating adjacent structures or organs, for example, uterus, prostate gland, seminal glands, vagina, or urine bladder. Understaging of nonresectable carcinoma may occur due to severe stenosis. In such cases, small-caliber instruments may prove helpful.

Important for the surgeon is delineation of the tumor-free margins, both proximal and distal, from the primary tumor site. Moreover, lymph nodes adjacent to and distant from the edge of the tumor should be examined carefully. In this manner, radical tumor resection and radical lymph node dissection can be performed. This is of utmost importance considering the high incidence of local recurrence.

In cases of nonsurgical treatment with laser photocoagulation or irradiation, the depth of tumor infiltration before and after treatment should be measured carefully. Documentation can be made after therapy regarding tumor size and extent. Tissue changes after treatment, however, may simulate the remnants of malignancy. Therefore, multiple biopsies or EUS-guided cytology should be performed to confirm the diagnosis of malignancy. In some centers, the strategy of treatment is planned on the basis of EUS findings. A T1 carcinoma without evidence of lymph node involvement can be treated with transanal microsurgery or laser photocoagulation. These therapeutic procedures can also be performed in high-risk patients undergoing surgery for T2 carcinoma. In our series, the incidence of lymph node involvement in T1 carcinoma was 11%, paradoxically in T2 0% (none of 19 cases), in T3 53%, and in T4 60%. There was no correlation between the size of lymph nodes and the presence of metastatic involvement.[12]

Suprarectal Colon

Case Report

In a 70-year-old man with ulcerative colitis, a sigmoid carcinoma was found in the involved segment during the follow-up period of 10 years. EUS showed a circumscribed hypoechoic tumor with tiny penetration through the muscle layer into the subserosal layer. No lymph node involvement was found. Low anterior resection was performed. The EUS findings were confirmed by the histology of the resected specimen.

RECURRENT TUMORS

Local tumor recurrence is one of the most common complications after surgical therapy. Local recurrence is defined as the reappearance of a hypoechoic intramural or transmural echo pattern adjacent to the previous site of disease after radical surgical or complete endoscopic removal of tumor. The diagnosis, however, should be confirmed by biopsy or EUS-guided cytology. Recurrence in this definition should be distinguished from the occurrence of residual tumors left behind after incomplete excision. Pelvic recurrence of colorectal cancer is defined as tumor reappearance in the pelvic floor without fixation in the pelvic walls.

Recurrent tumors can be incorporated into the TNM classification. Both the long-term follow-up of patients showing local recurrence and the staging of recurrent tumors are essential for the evaluation of therapeutic results. The technique of EUS investigation is similar to that described in previous sections. Thus, an initial EUS should be performed following surgery as a basis for comparison with subsequent EUS findings during long-term follow-up; this permits findings related to the carcinomatous recurrences to be distinguished from post-surgical artifact. EUS-guided cytology or biopsy is recommended for confirmation of the diagnosis.

Esophagus

After distal esophageal resection for carcinoma, a recurrent tumor appears as a hypoechoic pattern adjacent to the anastomosis. An ulcerative lesion or a mass with normal, overlying mucosa may be seen bulging into the lumen. In cases in which the biopsy result is negative, EUS-guided cytological puncture should be performed to establish the diagnosis.[6] This is important because lymph node metastasis adjacent to the anastomosis may show a similar echo pattern with those of tumor recurrence. The prognosis of such diseases, however, is generally worse.

In our small series, we found advanced stages of recurrent carcinoma. At Memorial Sloan-Kettering center, Lightdale et al. reported on the sensitivity of EUS of 95% in the detection of recurrent cancer.[35] Descriptions of such carcinomas should add the prefix "r" to the TNM classification. Differentiation between surgical changes and recurrent tumor tissue can be made on the basis of progression in size and extent and changes in echo pattern. The depth of tumor infiltration can be staged according to the TNM classification.

Case Report

In a 78-year-old man who had undergone distal esophageal resection for carcinoma, endoscopy following oral administration of barium revealed a polypoid lesion at the anastomosis. Results of multiple endoscopically guided biopsies were negative for carcinoma. CT scan uncovered no abnormality. EUS was performed with the latest commercially available echoendoscope, equipped with a biopsy channel for cytological puncture and an adjustable frequency of 7.5 or 12 MHz. A hypoechoic transmural echo pattern was found at the anastomosis bulging into the lumen. EUS-guided cytological puncture was performed. Malignant cells were found consistent with the diagnosis of locally recurrent carcinoma.

Stomach

Locally recurrent tumor can occur after partial or total resection of the stomach. The feature and local extent of the malignancy show an echo pattern similar to that previously described. A surgical approach is usually unfavorable because of the advanced stage and the poor prognosis.

Linitis plastica confirmed to be nonresectable at surgery may be treated with radiotherapy or chemotherapy, or both. EUS is accurate for the documentation of response to therapy. Noneffective treatment is suggested on ultrasound by the absence of reduction in abnormalities in terms of both mural and nodal involvement. Partial remission is defined as reduction in mural and nodal abnormality. After partial remission, surgical resection can be performed. In these cases, the prefix "Y" should be added to the TNM classification.

Residual tumor may occasionally be found, particularly in cases of linitis plastica, when the proximal edge of tumors has not been adequately removed. The most common cause of such incomplete resection is submucosal infiltration, which is usually covered with intact mucosa. This may not be defined at endoscopy or biopsy, and even at surgery such a submucosal abnormality may not be palpable or visible on macroscopic inspection. In these cases the prefix "R" should be added to the TNM classification.

Case Report

In a 64-year-old man after a previous partial proximal gastrectomy for carcinoma (pT2N1), endoscopy revealed a narrowing of the anastomosis. The results of endoscopic biopsy were negative for carcinoma. EUS was performed after endoscopic dilation of the stenosis and showed a semicircular transtumoral hypoechoic tumor covered with smooth mucosa. Lymph node metastasis was also found. This anatomical site is known as one of predilection for metastasis.

Pancreas and Ampulla of Vater

Recurrent pancreatic carcinoma is more frequent than intestinal carcinoma because of its highly malignant nature. Malignant carcinomas may be found locally or spreading diffusely in the remnants of the organ.

Carcinoma of the ampulla of Vater has a more favorable prognosis. Local recurrent carcinomas may be found adjacent to the previous site of disease or diffusely in the rest of the pancreatic parenchyma. After Whipple's resection, the body and tail of the pancreas can be imaged by filling the stomach with water. The pancreatic duct should be visualized clearly to predict the functioning of the pancreaticojejunal anastomosis. The jejunopancreatic anastomosis can be visualized using the pancreatic duct as a landmark. This technique appears promising because of the ability to image ductural and parenchymal abnormality without cannulation of the duct and because of the lack of disturbances in images after surgical treatment.

Case Report

A 43-year-old woman with obstructive jaundice was referred for ERCP. Ampullary carcinoma was confirmed by biopsy with dilatation of the common bile duct and pancreatic duct. Preoperative EUS revealed a transmural ampullary carcinoma with penetration into the common bile duct and pancreas. The depth of infiltration was less than 2 cm. Multiple lymph nodes were found. Histology revealed a pT2N1 carcinoma. Additional radiotherapy was done 2 years after surgery. Multiple lymph node metastases were found associated with obstructive jaundice. The patient died due to the widespread malignant disease.

Extrahepatic Bile Duct

The investigation after Whipple's resection for extrahepatic bile duct carcinoma resembles that for ampullopancreatic carcinoma. Local recurrence may be expected adjacent to the anastomosis. The long-term prognosis tends to be unfavorable despite a low incidence of distant metastasis.

Successful assessment after proximal bile duct surgery depends on the previous surgical procedure. In the case of extended left hepatic lobe resection, the remnants of the organ may not be imaged because of the inability to reach the target lesion, however, right hepatic lobe resection may provide imaging of the remnants or organ. Local recurrence appears as a hypoechoic abnormality with dilation of the corresponding bile duct. Regional lymph node metastasis is often detected. After irradiation, it is possible to image thickening of the bile duct wall, periductular hyperechoic fibrosis, and dilation of the adjacent hepatic ducts. Distinction between irradiation damage and local tumor recurrence is difficult on EUS except if pre-treatment EUS is performed. Therefore, cytological puncture or brush cytology should be advocated.

Case Report

A 33-year-old patient with painless jaundice was referred for ERCP. Proximal extrahepatic bile duct obstruction strongly suspect for Klatskin tumor was found. EUS revealed a hypoechoic transductal echo pattern at the bifurcation, with some multifocal intraductal spread. Tumor resection with extended liver resection was performed. Histology of the resected specimen confirmed the EUS diagnosis (pT2N0). Three years after resection multiple recurrent tumors were found, with obstructed jaundice. The patient died of recurrent carcinomas.

Colon and Rectum

After low anterior resection for carcinoma locally recurrent tumors may be found adjacent to the anastomosis. Early stages of recurrent tumors can be resected, however, advanced-stage carcinomas should undergo surgery only when complicated by obstruction. The long-term prognosis is nevertheless dubious. Polypoid lesions adjacent to the anastomosis after resection may be caused by granulomatous inflammation due to reaction to clip material (foreign body reaction). An intra- and transmural hypoechoic echo pattern may appear on ultrasound, which may simulate the presence of local recurrence. Biopsy and/or EUS-guided cytology is required for establishing the final diagnosis. In cases of submucosal recurrent carcinoma covered with smooth overlying mucosa, endoscopy and EUS may suggest the presence of leiomyomas or postsurgical tissue changes. Biopsy using a giant biopsy forceps and EUS-guided cytology should be performed. In cases of intramural recurrent carcinoma (T1 or T2 carcinoma) without evidence of lymph node involvement, local resection can be considered. Transanal resection of rectal carcinoma has recently become available in some centers.

Case Report

In a 64-year-old patient 2 years after radical endoscopic removal of sigmoid polyps, a small bulging lesion of biopsy confirmed malignancy was found during follow-up endoscopy. EUS revealed a hypoechoic intramural infiltration penetrating the muscularis propria without evidence of lymph node involvement. Local surgical resection was performed. The diagnosis of EUS was confirmed by histology.

Case Report

A 67-year-old woman with rectal bleeding was referred for sigmoidoscopy. Rectal carcinoma was found. Preoperative EUS revealed a T3 carcinoma without evidence of lymph node metastases. Low anterior resection was performed. Histology confirmed the EUS findings. A narrowing of the anastomosis was found 6 months after surgery. Biopsy was negative for carcinoma. EUS revealed a semicircular infiltration with an extensive presacral mass strongly suspected to be a metastasis. Metastatic lymph nodes were also found adjacent to the iliac vessels. EUS-guided cytology and biopsy confirmed the diagnosis of recurrent carcinoma. Thus, the diagnosis was rT3N3.

RESIDUAL TUMOR

Residual tumor is defined as a remnant of malignant disease after endoscopic or surgical resection, laser photocoagulation, thermophotocoagulation, radiotherapy, or chemotherapy. Pretherapeutic EUS documentation is essential to select appropriate treatment. Follow-up EUS investigation is mandatory to document the response to treatment. Examination of tissue is obligatory for establishing the diagnosis. Indirect diagnosis may be suggested in nonradical resected carcinomatous tissue by assessing resected margins and showing carcinomatous infiltration. The final diagnosis, however, should be confirmed by biopsy or EUS-guided cytological puncture. Clinically residual carcinoma is often diagnosed in the case of linitis plastica (scirrhous carcinoma) because submucosal infiltration may not be seen at surgery. Thus, nonradical resection of carcinoma may be performed erroneously because submucosal growth of carcinoma is not seen at surgery. Surgical reintervention or irradiation may become necessary.

In biliopancreatic surgery, nonradical tumor resection is found more often in Klatskin tumors than in distal common bile duct carcinomas. EUS may be helpful for diagnosing the carcinomatous remnant when the target of interest can be visualized by this means. A special surgical technique for performing the biliodigestive anastomosis is necessary to allow the instrument through the loop to the site of the biliodigestive anastomosis.

Intraluminal Radiotherapy (After Loading, Brachytherapy)

In cases of intraluminal irradiation (in addition to extracorporal radiotherapy) of esophageal carcinoma, EUS is the imaging technique of choice for the documentation of response to therapy.[17] Reduction in the depth of tumor infiltration and in the size and number of involved lymph nodes is consistent with partial remission. Total remission is defined as the disappearance of mural and nodal abnormalities. Thickening of the involved esophageal wall, however, is often present due to fibrosis after irradiation. In cases of negative biopsy results, EUS-guided cytology may be helpful for establishing the diagnosis of carcinoma. The prognosis tends to be unfavorable due to the presence of deep penetration into the adjacent structures or the presence of celiac lymph node metastases or liver dissemination. In such cases, intraluminal radiotherapy may also be contraindicated. In patients with unresectable tumors or those who were inoperable because of their poor general condition, intraluminal irradiation may become an alternative treatment. In our series involving 63 cases with inoperable esophageal carcinoma, staging was incomplete in 31 of 63 cases because of the tight stenosis which cannot be passed with the instrument or the difficulty in imaging the celiac lymph nodes by using nonoptic echoprobe. During follow-up, reduction of tumor thickness and number of lymph node abnormalities could be accurately documented. The median survival was 10.4 months. Patients with fewer than five metastatic lymph nodes had a significantly better survival rate. Paradoxically, patients with more extended intraluminal tumor showed a significantly better survival rate than those with less tumor extent. Survival correlated with initial number and size of the lymph nodes.

Laser Photocoagulation

Endoscopy is accurate for evaluation of the entire mucosal (intraluminal) extent of carcinoma before and after laser treatment. The intrasubmucosal extent of disease, however, cannot be assessed. EUS is thus essential for accurate documentation of laser treatment. A remnant of carcinoma appears readily as a hypoechoic submucosal echo pattern, which may be erroneously diagnosed by endoscopy as a scarring effect after laser therapy.[36] Distinction between irradiation damages and recurrent carcinomas is not always possible by endoscopy and EUS. Thus, routine EUS-guided cytology is recommended. Recently, EUS has been reported to be helpful in selecting and monitoring the effect of photodynamic therapy for esophageal carcinoma.

Case Report

In an 80-year-old man with an early gastric carcinoma (ulcerative type), laser treatment was performed due to the patient's poor general condition for surgery. During follow-up, the intramural hypoechoic echo pattern directly adjacent to the ulceration showed no changes in extent, size, or anatomical localization. Moreover, no nodal abnormalities were found. EUS-guided cytology showed no malignant cells. The EUS findings and clinical status of the patient indicated a steady stage.

Photodynamic Therapy

Photodynamic therapy (PTD) is suitable for the treatment of early gastroesophageal cancer. In case of esophageal cancer, only patients staged by EUS as T1 N0 should be treated with PTD. Recently, endoscopy and EUS have been reported to be accurate in monitoring the response to PTD.[38] These authors concluded that endoscopy remained necessary to detect recurrence as EUS missed most superficial recurrences and there was a risk of making a false-positive diagnosis after radiotherapy. EUS was necessary to detect recurrence and to help clinicians in deciding whether to undertake further treatment. Most importantly, normal or unchanged EUS pattern with negative biopsy during follow-up was a strong argument for prolonged remission.

NATURAL HISTORY AND SURVEILLANCE OF EARLY CANCER

The natural history of gastric cancer and esophageal cancer has been frequently reported in Japan and China. An early cancer needs a period of time to develop to an advanced cancer. Recently, high-risk areas for esophageal cancers such as northern China (Lin-Xian), northern Iran, the central Asian republics of the former Soviet Union, and South Africa have been reported. In some of these regions, the mortality rate for esophageal cancer almost surpassed 20%. Endoscopic surveys in high-risk and low-risk populations for esophageal cancer in China were carried out in 1987.[39] Recently, endoscopy has been proven to be helpful in the detection of squamous dysplasia and early esophageal cancer.[40] The accuracy was 81% if biopsy was undertaken every 4 cm and additional specimens taken from all visually abnormal areas. The accuracy would have been 91% if only visible target lesions—friability, focal red area, erosion, plaque, and nodule—had been sampled. Dawsey et al concluded that for surveillance in this high-risk population, random biopsy specimens may be unnecessary. Sampling the target lesions described appears sufficient to detect nearly all invasive cancer and most dysplasia. Recently, an ongoing study has been undertaken in this high-risk area using endoscopy with mucosal staining and EUS.

REFERENCES

1. Hermanek P, Sobin LH (eds): *TNM Classification of Malignant Tumours,* ed 4. New York, Springer, 1987.
2. Sobin LH, Hermanek P, Hutter RP: TNM classification of malignant tumours. *Cancer* 61:2310–2314, 1988.
3. Spiessl B, Beahrs OH, Hermanek P, et al (eds): *TNM Atlas,* ed 3. New York, Springer, 1989.
4. Tio TL, Tytgat GNJ: *Atlas of Transintestinal Ultrasonography.* Aalsmeer, The Netherlands, Mur-Kostverloren, 1986.
5. Tio TL, Tytgat GNJ: Endoscopic ultrasonography in the assessment of intra- and transmural infiltration of tumours in the esophagus and papilla of vater and in the detection of extraesophageal lesions. *Endoscopy* 16:203–210, 1984.
6. Tio TL, Cohen P, Coene PP, et al: Preoperative TNM classification of esophageal carcinoma by endoscopy and computed tomography. *Gastroenterology* 96:1478–1486, 1989.
7. Tio TL, Schouwink MH, Cikot R, et al: Preoperative TNM classification of gastric carcinoma by endosonography in comparison with the pathological TNM system: A prospective study of 72 cases. *Hepato-Gastroenterology* 36:51–56, 1989.
8. Tio TL, Coene PPLO, Schouwink MH, et al: Esophagogastric carcinoma: Preoperative TNM classification with endosonography. *Radiology* 73:411–417, 1989.
9. Tio TL, Tytgat GNJ, Cikot RJLM, et al: Ampullopancreatic carcinoma: Preoperative TNM classification with endosonography. *Radiology* 175:455–461, 1990.
10. Yasuda K, Mukai H, Fujimoto S, et al: The diagnosis of pancreatic cancer by endoscopic ultrasonography. *Gastrointest Endosc* 34:1–8, 1988.
11. Tio TL, Cheng J, Sars PRA, et al: Preoperative TNM classification of extrahepatic bile duct carcinoma by endosonography. *Gastroenterology* 10:1351–1361, 1991.
12. Tio TL, Coene PPLO, van Delden O, et al: Colorectal carcinoma: Preoperative TNM classification by endosonography. *Radiology* 179:165–170, 1991.
13. Tio TL, Tytgat GNJ: Endoscopic ultrasonography of normal and pathologic upper gastrointestinal wall structure. Comparison of studies in vitro and in vivo. *Scand J Gastroenterol 21* (suppl 123):27–33, 1986.
14. Kimmey MB, Martin RW, Haggit C, et al: Histologic correlates of gastrointestinal ultrasound images. *Gastroenterology* 96:433–441, 1989.
15. Grimm H, Binnmoeller KF, Soehendra N: Ultrasonic esophagoprobe (prototype 1). *Gastrointest Endosc* 38:490–493, 1992.
16. Tio TL, Tytgat GNJ: Endoscopic ultrasonography in analysing periintestinal lymnode abnormality. *Scand J Gastroenterol 21* 123:158–163, 1986.
17. Tio TL, Blank LECM, Weijers OB, et al: Staging and prognosis using endosonography in patients with inoperable esophageal carcinoma treated with combined irradiation. *Gastrointest Endosc* (in press).
18. Lightdale CJ: Endoscopic ultrasonography in diagnosing, staging and follow-up of esophageal and gastric cancer. *Endoscopy* 24 1:297–303, 1992.
19. Tio TL, Maas JJ, Colin EM, et al: Endosonography in diagnosing and staging diffuse gastric wall abnormalities. DDW 1992, Abstract 2520.
20. Morson BC: *Colour Atlas of Gastrointestinal Pathology.* Oxford, Miller, 1988.
21. Tio TL, Sie LH, Verbeek PCM, et al: Endosonography in diagnosing and staging duodenal villous adenoma. *Gut* 33:567–568, 1992.
22. Cubilla AL, Fortner J, Fitzgerald J: Lymph node involvement in carcinoma of the head of the pancreas area. *Cancer* 41:880–887, 1978.

23. Tio TL: Endoscopic Ultrasonography. In Trede M, Carter DC (eds.): *Surgery of the Pancreas*. Churchill Livingstone, 1993, pp 111–119.

24. Nagai H, Kuroda A, Moroika Y: Lymphatic and local spread of T1 and T2 pancreatic cancer: A study of autopsy material. *Ann Surg* 204:65–71, 1986.

25. Tio TL, Luiken GJHM: Endosonography in the clinical TNM staging of gastric cancer. Presented at the 4th general meeting of WHO collaborating centers for primary prevention, diagnosis and treatment of gastric cancer and the 9th WHO international workshop. Tokyo, June 5–7, 1990.

26. Snady H, Cooperman A, Siegel JH: Endoscopic ultrasonography compared with computed tomography and ERCP in patients with obstructive jaundice and small pancreatic mass. *Gastrointest Endosc* 38:27–34, 1992.

27. Tio TL, Sie LH, Tytgat GNJ: Endosonography and cytology in diagnosing and staging pancreatic body and tail carcinoma. *Dig Dis Sci* 38:59–64, 1993.

28. Tio TL, Mulder, Eggink WF: Endosonography in staging early carcinoma of the ampulla of vater. *Gastroenterology* 102:1392–1395, 1992.

29. Altenmeier WA, Gall EA, Zinninger MM, et al: Sclerosing carcinoma of the major mitrahepatic bile ducts. *Arch Surg* 75:450–460, 1956.

30. Klatskin G: Adenocarcinoma of the hepatic duct at its bifurcation within porta hepatis: An unusual tumor with distinctive clinical and pathological features. *AM J Med* 38:241–256, 1965.

31. Tio TL: *Atlas of Endosonography.* Lake Success, NY, Interactive Video Laser Disc Program Olympus, 1993.

32. Morita K, Nakazawa S, Kimoto E, et al: Gallbladder Disease. In Kawai K (ed): *Endoscopic Ultrasonography in Gastroenterology* Tokyo, Igaku-Shoin, 1988, p 87.

33. Tio TL: Endosonography of Colorectal Disease. *Endoscopy* 2, 1992, pp 99–109.

34. Hulsman FJ, Tio TL, Mathus-Vliegen E, et al: Colorectal villous adenoma: Transrectal US for screening of invasive malignancy. *Radiology* 185:193–196, 1992.

35. Lightdale CJ, Botet JF: Esophageal carcinoma: Preoperative staging and evaluation of anantomotic recurrence. *Gastrointest Endosc* 36(Suppl 1):11–16, 1990.

36. Yasuda K, Kiyota K, Nakajima M, et al: Fundamentals of endoscopic laser therapy for GI tumors—new aspects with endoscopic ultrasonography (EUS). *Endoscopy* 19(Suppl 1):2–6, 1987.

37. Souquet JC, Napoleon B, Pujol B, et al: Endosonographic-guided treatment of esophageal carcinoma. *Endoscopy* 24:324–328, 1992.

38. Souquet JC, Napoleon B, Sibille A, et al: Echoendoscopy in the follow-up of uT1N0 esophageal squamous carcinoma treated by photodynamic therapy. DDW 1994, Abstract 1378.

39. Yang GR, Qui SL: Endoscopic surveys in high-risk and low-risk population of esophageal cancer in China with special reference to precursors of esophageal cancer. *Endoscopy* 19:91–95, 1987.

40. Dawsey SM, Wang GQ, Weinstein WM, et al: Squamous dysplasia and early esophageal cancer in the linxian region of China: distinctive endoscopic lesions 105:1333–1340, 1993.

BIBLIOGRAPHY

1. Glaser F, Kuntz C, Schlag P, et al: Endorectal ultrasound for control of preoperative radiotherapy of rectal cancer. *Ann Surg* 217:64–71, 1993.

2. Hermanek P, Guggenmoos-Hilzman I, Gall FP: Prognostic factors in rectal carcinoma. A contribution to the further development of tumor classification. *Dis Colon Rectum* 32:593–599, 1989.

3. Rosch T, Braig C, Gain T, et al: Staging of pancreatic and ampullary carcinoma by endoscopic ultrasonography. *Gastroenterology* 102:188–199, 1992.

4. Sherman CD, Calman KC, Eckhardt S (eds): *Manual of Clinical Oncology,* Ed 4. New York, Springer-Verlag, 1987.

5. Sobin LH, Kos PR: Radiology and the new TNM classification of tumors: The future. *Radiology* 176:1–4.

6. Takeda M: *Atlas of Diagnostic Gastrointestinal Cytology.* New York, Igaku-Shoin, 1983.

7. Tio TL: Endoscopic ultrasonography in the detection and staging of intramural and extramural lesions in the upper gastrointestinal tract. In Pfeifel, Hildebrandt (eds.) *Endosonography in Surgery, Gastroenterology, Urology and Gynecology.* New York, Springer-Verlag, 1990.

8. Tio TL: *Endosonography in Gastroenterology.* New York, Springer-Verlag, 1988.

9. Tio TL, Tytgat GNJ: Endoscopic ultrasonography in the preoperative staging of biliopancreatic carcinoma. In Lygidakis NJ, Tytgat GNJ (eds): *Hepatobiliary and Pancreatic Malignancy.* New York, Thieme, 1989, pp 66–78.

10. Tio TL, Wijers OB, Sars PRA, et al: Preoperative TNM classification of proximal extrahepatic bile duct carcinoma by endosonography *Sem Liver Dis* 10:114–120, 1990.

Figure 1

A.

An Olympus commercially available echoendoscope (EU M3) with an echoprobe (E) attached to a side-viewing duodenoscope and a sclerosing needle (N) passing through the biopsy channel.

B.

An Olympus prototype videoechoendoscope (VUM3) with an echoprobe (E) smaller than the diameter of the endoscope.

C.

An Olympus prototype echoendoscope (EUM4) with an echoprobe (E) smaller than the diameter of an endoscope and elevator (EL) for maneuvering the needle (N) or catheter during cytological procedures.

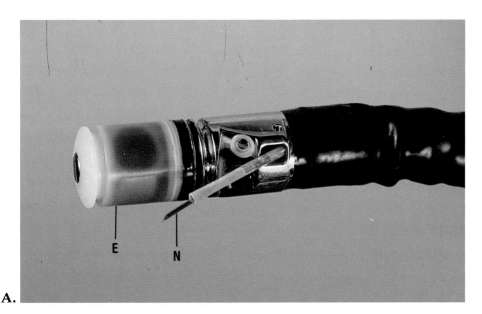

A.

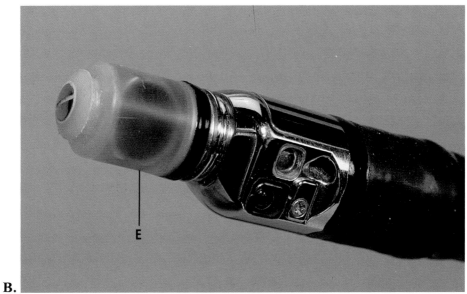

B.

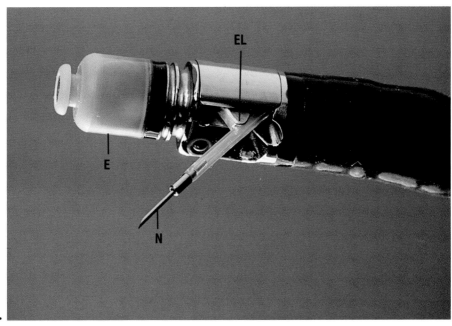

C.

Figure 2

A.
An Aloka flexible nonoptic echo instrument with an echoprobe (E) attached to a flexible small-caliber shaft.

B.
An Olympus catheter echoprobe (E) without a balloon at its tip passing through the instrumental channel of a large-caliber gastroscope for endoscopic-guided endosonography.

C.
A commercially available catheter echoprobe (E) with a balloon (B) attached at its tip.

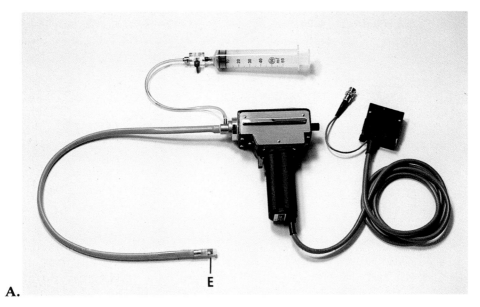

A.

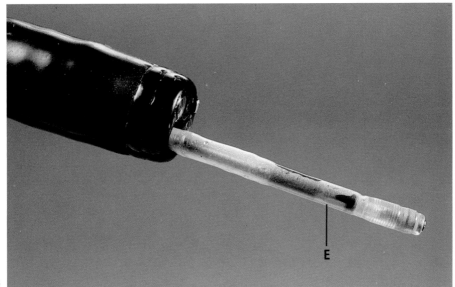

B.

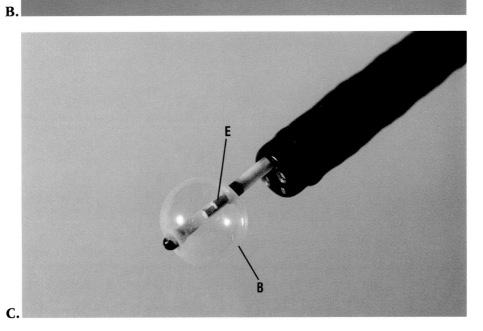

C.

Figure 3

A.
A cross section through the cervical esophagus shows laterally the carotid arteries (C) and the jugular vein (J), ventrally the trachea reverberation (arrows) of hyperechoic pattern, and dorsally the vertebra (V).

B.
A cross section through the midesophagus shows the aortic arch (AR) on the left and the azygos vein (AV) at the contralateral side communicating with the superior vena cava (SVC).

C.
A cross section through the lower esophagus shows the descending aorta (AO) on the left, the pulmonary artery (PA) ventrally, and the vertebra (V) dorsally.

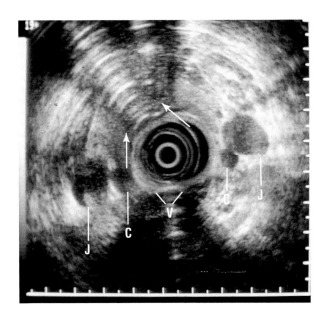

A.

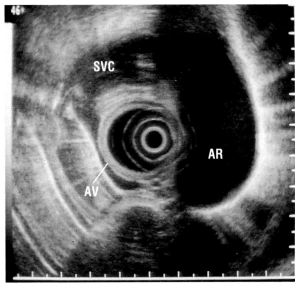

B.

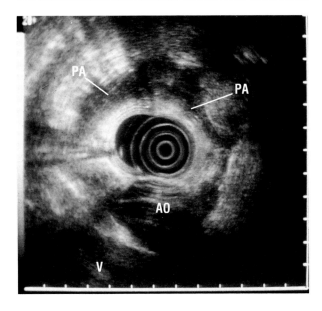

C.

Figure 4

A.
A cross section through the subcardial stomach shows the celiac trunk (CT) with the bifurcation of the splenic artery (SA) and hepatic artery (HA).

B.
A cross section through the midcorpus of the stomach shows the splenic vein (SV), renal vein (RV), pancreas (P), left kidney (LK), and spleen (SP). Note that the renal vein is located dorsally and parallel to the splenic vein and renal artery (RA).

C.
Another cross section shows the relationship between the splenic vein (SV), renal vein (RV), and the renal artery (RA). SH = splenic hilum, SP = spleen, LK = left kidney.

A.

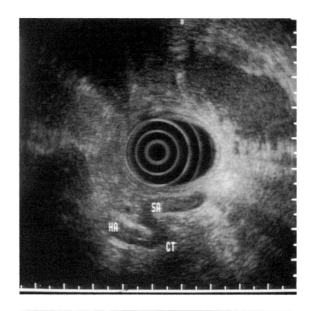

B.

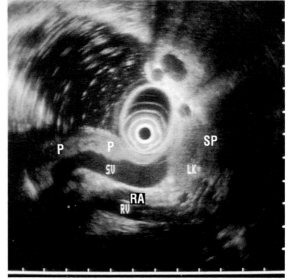

C.

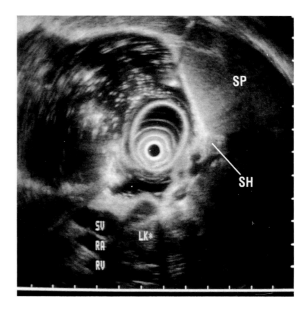

Figure 5

A.
A longitudinal section shows the common bile duct (CBD) parallel and ventral to the portal vein (PV). RL = right lobe of liver, P = pancreas.

B.
Another longitudinal section comparable to ERCP images shows the (dilated) common bile duct (CBD), common hepatic duct (CHD), and gallbladder (GB). Note the location of the portal vein (PV). P = pancreas, PD = pancreatic duct.

C.
This longitudinal section shows that the splenic vein (SV) runs from the splenic hilum (SH) along the dorsal surface from the pancreas to the spleno-portal confluence (CF) and joins the superior mesenteric vein (SMV) to form the portal vein (PV) to the hilum of the liver (LH).

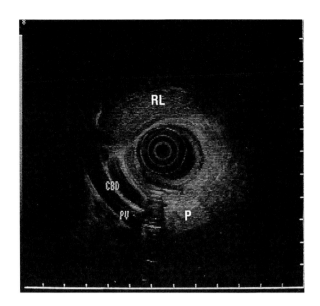

A.

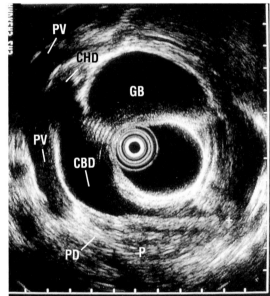

B.

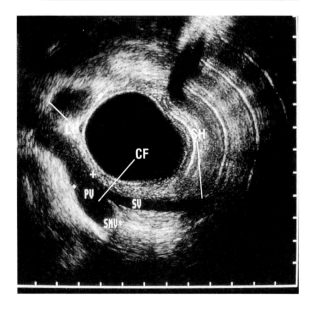

C.

Figure 6

A.
A cross section through the suprapapillary duodenum shows the pancreatic duct (PD), splenic vein (SV) and superior mesenteric artery (SMA), aorta (AO), and vena cava (VC).

B.
A cross section through the infrabulbar duodenum shows the uncinate process (UP) adjacent to the superior mesenteric vein (SMV), superior mesenteric artery (SMA) and the aorta (AO). Note the portal vein (PV) and the left renal vein (RV).

C.
A corresponding CT shows the pancreas (P), aorta (AO), vena cava (VC), renal vein (RV), superior mesenteric artery (SMA), splenic vein (SV), and gallbladder (GB).

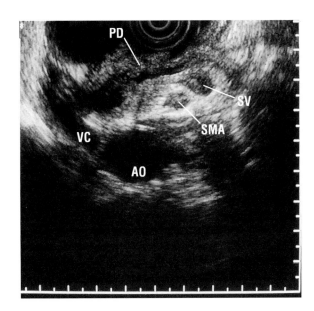

A.

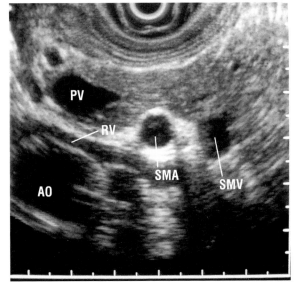

B.

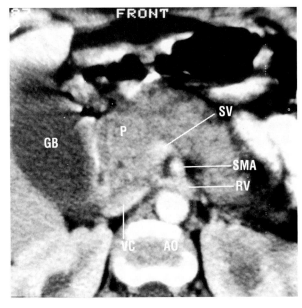

C.

Figure 7

A.

A cross section immediately adjacent to the papilla of Vater shows the aorta (AO), vena cava (VC), arteria mesenterica superior (AMS), pancreas (P), and splenic vein (SV). PV = portal vein, CBD = common bile duct.

B.

This cross section shows the papilla (ampulla) of Vater with the adjacent pancreatic duct (PD) and common bile duct (CBD). P = pancreatic parenchyma.

C.

A cross section distal from the ampulla shows the inferior vena cava (IVC), aorta (AO), vertebra (V), vena mesenterica superior (VMS), main pancreatic duct (PD), and uncinate process of the pancreas. T = small hypoechoic tumor in the uncinate process.

A.

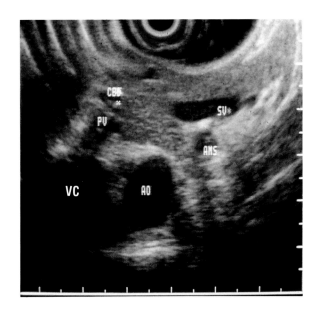

B.

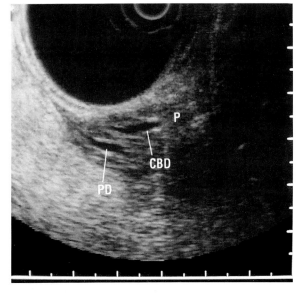

C.

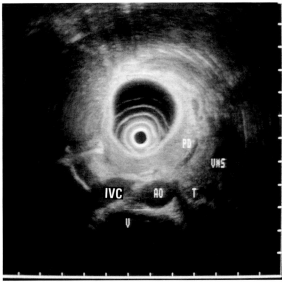

Figure 8 A 71-year-old man was referred for staging of esophageal carcinoma.

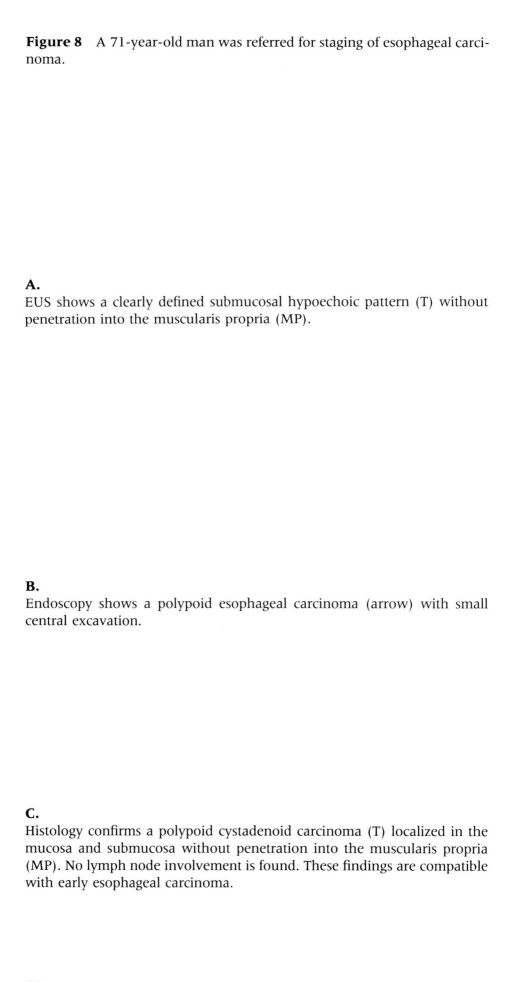

A.
EUS shows a clearly defined submucosal hypoechoic pattern (T) without penetration into the muscularis propria (MP).

B.
Endoscopy shows a polypoid esophageal carcinoma (arrow) with small central excavation.

C.
Histology confirms a polypoid cystadenoid carcinoma (T) localized in the mucosa and submucosa without penetration into the muscularis propria (MP). No lymph node involvement is found. These findings are compatible with early esophageal carcinoma.

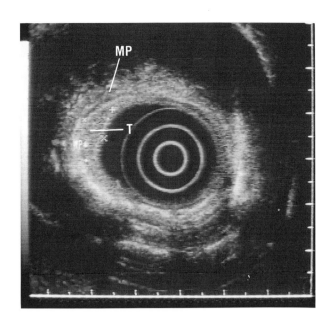

A.

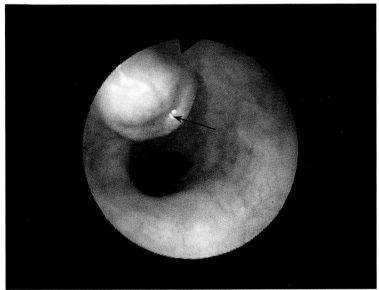

B.

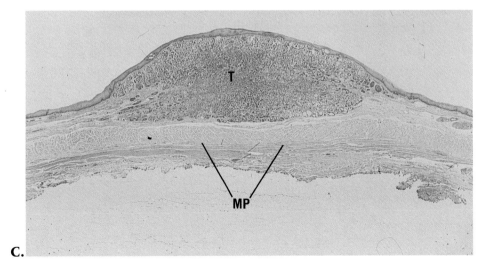

C.

Figure 9 A 64-year-old man with a carcinoma in the distal esophagus was referred for preoperative staging.

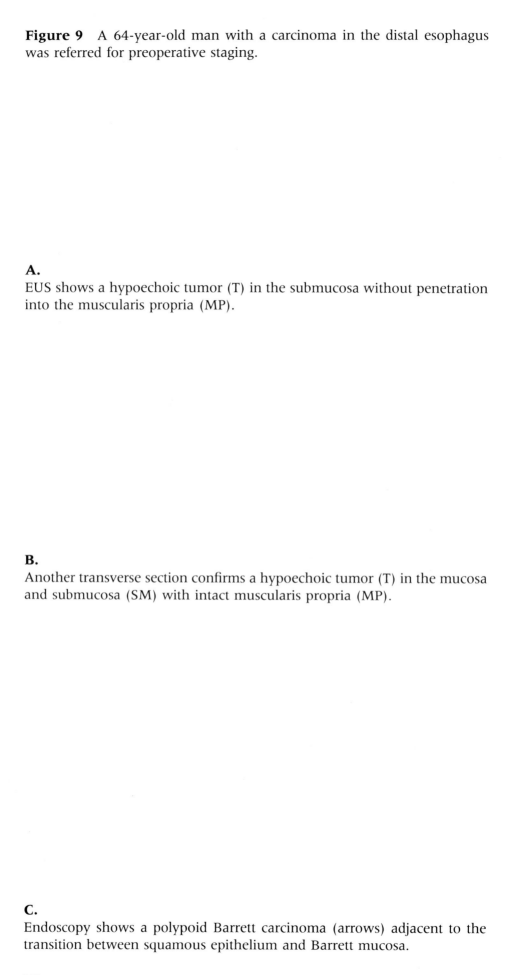

A.
EUS shows a hypoechoic tumor (T) in the submucosa without penetration into the muscularis propria (MP).

B.
Another transverse section confirms a hypoechoic tumor (T) in the mucosa and submucosa (SM) with intact muscularis propria (MP).

C.
Endoscopy shows a polypoid Barrett carcinoma (arrows) adjacent to the transition between squamous epithelium and Barrett mucosa.

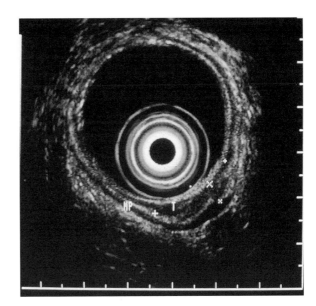

A.

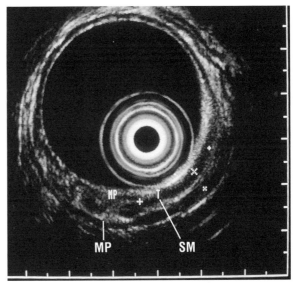

B.

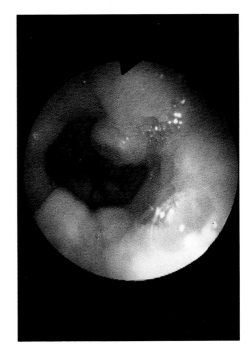

C.

Figure 10 A 63-year-old patient was referred for gastroscopy 2 weeks after coronary bypass surgery following myocardial infarction. A small ulcerative carcinoma in the distal esophagus was found. EUS was performed for staging.

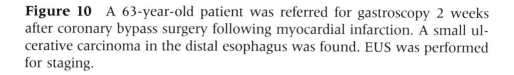

A.
EUS shows a hypoechoic tumor (T) in the mucosa and submucosa without penetration into the muscularis propria (MP). Surgery was recommended because of the early stage of the disease.

B.
Macrohistology confirms a carcinoma (T) in the submucosa without invasion into the muscularis propria (MP).

C.
Magnification section Barrett carcinoma (T).

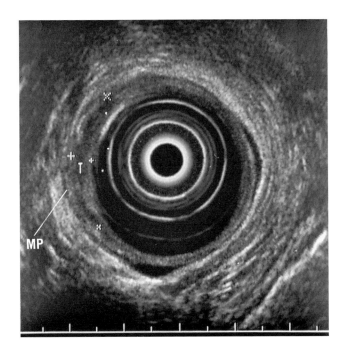

A.

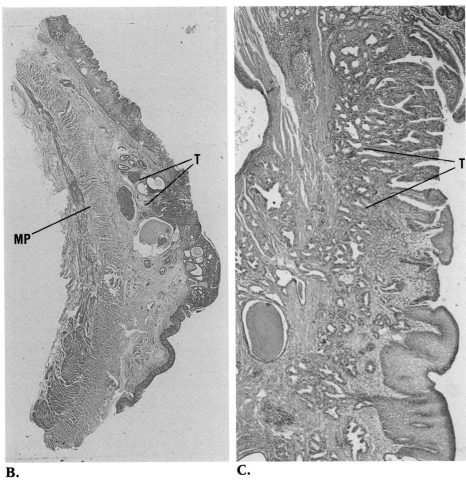

B.   **C.**

Figure 11   A 58-year-old woman was referred for endoscopy because of dysphagia. A small carcinoma was found in the midesophagus.

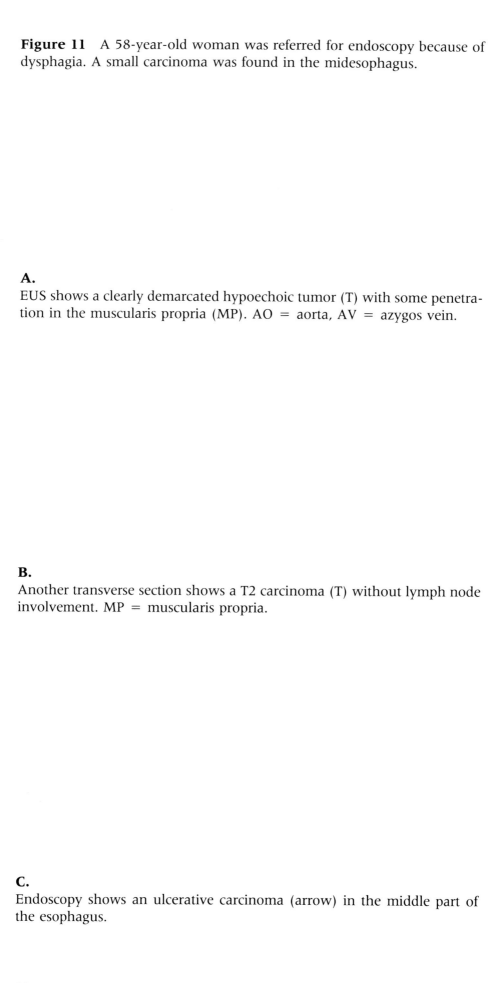

A.
EUS shows a clearly demarcated hypoechoic tumor (T) with some penetration in the muscularis propria (MP). AO = aorta, AV = azygos vein.

B.
Another transverse section shows a T2 carcinoma (T) without lymph node involvement. MP = muscularis propria.

C.
Endoscopy shows an ulcerative carcinoma (arrow) in the middle part of the esophagus.

A.

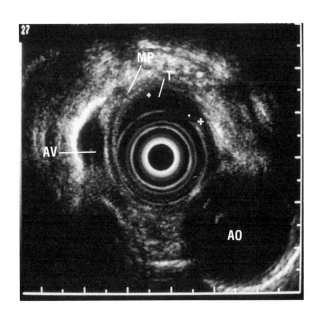

B.

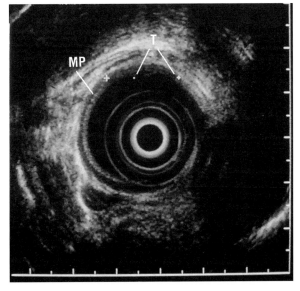

C.

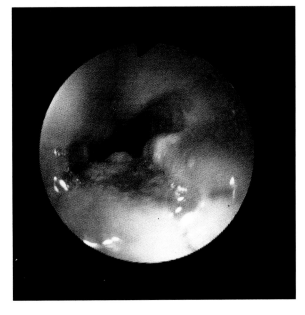

Figure 12 A 50-year-old woman was referred for endoscopy because of retrosternal pain and weight loss. Esophageal carcinoma was found in the midesophagus.

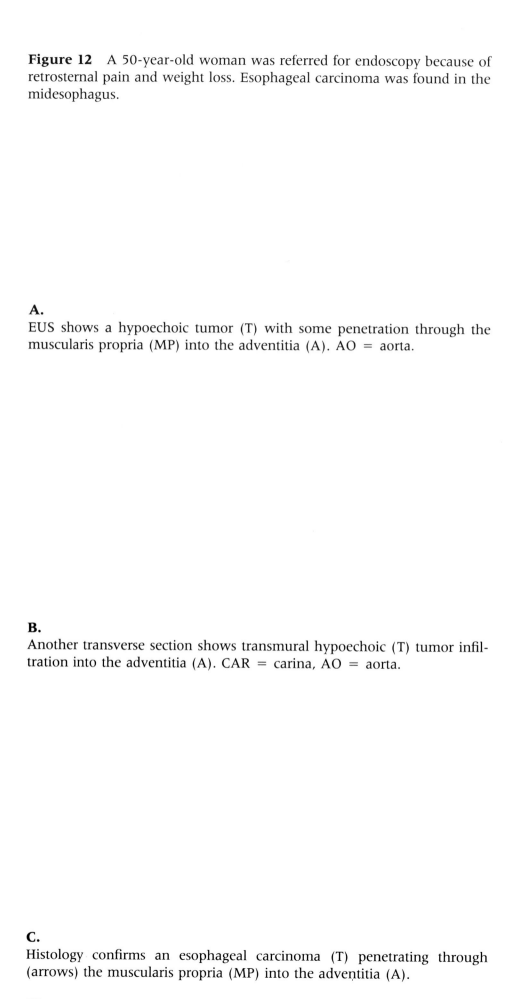

A.
EUS shows a hypoechoic tumor (T) with some penetration through the muscularis propria (MP) into the adventitia (A). AO = aorta.

B.
Another transverse section shows transmural hypoechoic (T) tumor infiltration into the adventitia (A). CAR = carina, AO = aorta.

C.
Histology confirms an esophageal carcinoma (T) penetrating through (arrows) the muscularis propria (MP) into the adventitia (A).

A.

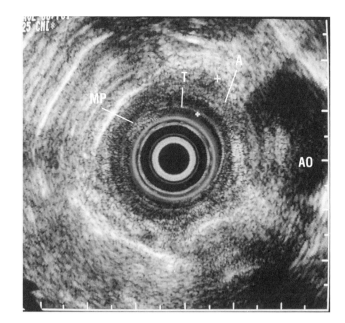

B.

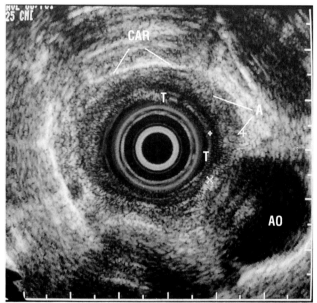

C.

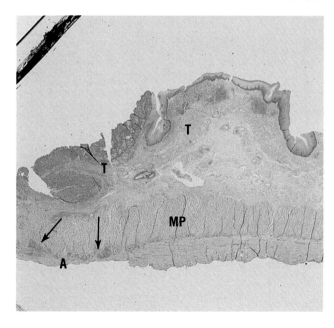

Figure 13 A 67-year-old man with alcoholic cirrhosis and esophageal varices was referred for gastroscopy. Esophageal carcinoma was found in the distal esophagus. Preoperative staging was performed with EUS and CT.

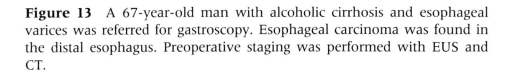

A.
EUS shows an ulcerative (U) hypoechoic tumor (T) with penetration into the muscularis propria (MP) at the contralateral side of the aorta (AO). AV = azygos vein.

B.
Corresponding CT shows wall thickening (T) at the contralateral side of the aorta (AO). C = contrast enhancement in the esophageal lumen.

C.
Histology of the resected specimen shows an ulcerative (U) with carcinoma (T) with polypoid margins (arrows) penetrating into the muscularis propria (MP).

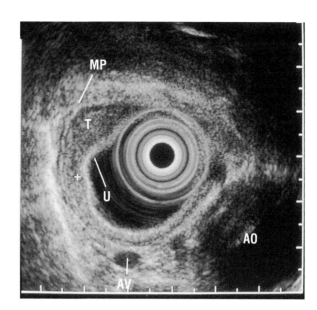

A.

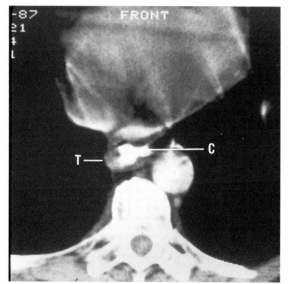

B.

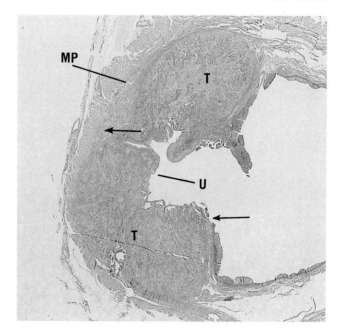

C.

Figure 14 A 68-year-old woman with esophageal carcinoma was referred for preoperative staging.

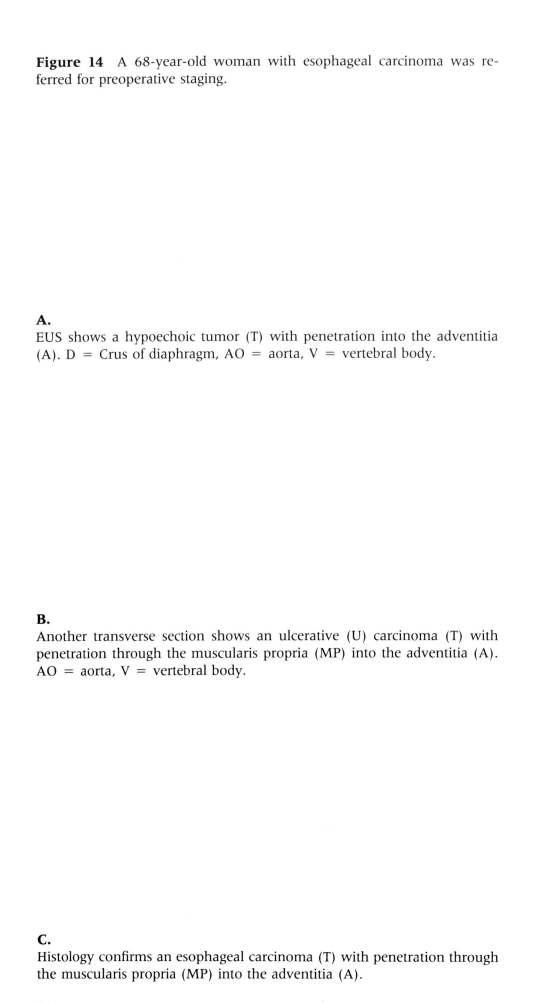

A.
EUS shows a hypoechoic tumor (T) with penetration into the adventitia (A). D = Crus of diaphragm, AO = aorta, V = vertebral body.

B.
Another transverse section shows an ulcerative (U) carcinoma (T) with penetration through the muscularis propria (MP) into the adventitia (A). AO = aorta, V = vertebral body.

C.
Histology confirms an esophageal carcinoma (T) with penetration through the muscularis propria (MP) into the adventitia (A).

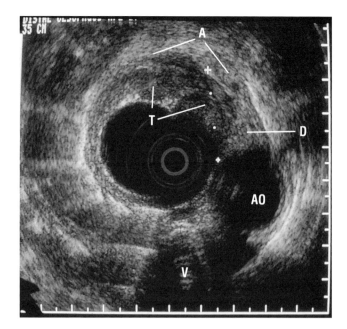

A.

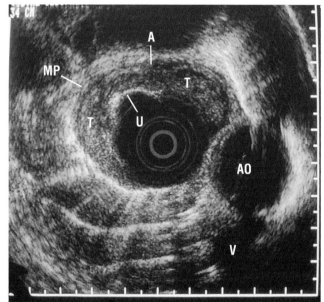

B.

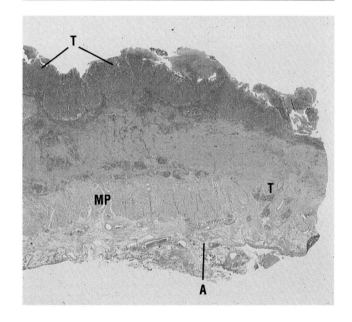

C.

Figure 15 A 61-year-old woman with esophageal carcinoma in the mid-esophagus was referred for preoperative staging.

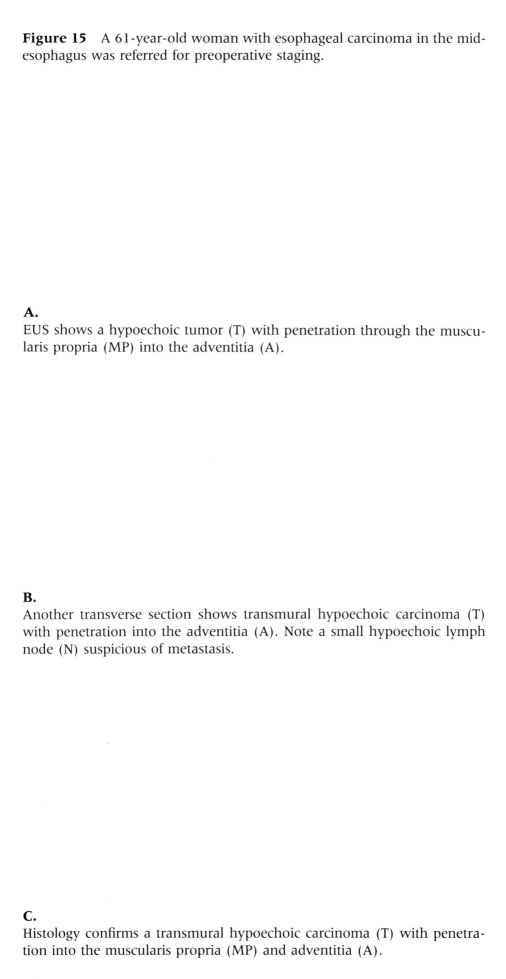

A.
EUS shows a hypoechoic tumor (T) with penetration through the muscularis propria (MP) into the adventitia (A).

B.
Another transverse section shows transmural hypoechoic carcinoma (T) with penetration into the adventitia (A). Note a small hypoechoic lymph node (N) suspicious of metastasis.

C.
Histology confirms a transmural hypoechoic carcinoma (T) with penetration into the muscularis propria (MP) and adventitia (A).

A.

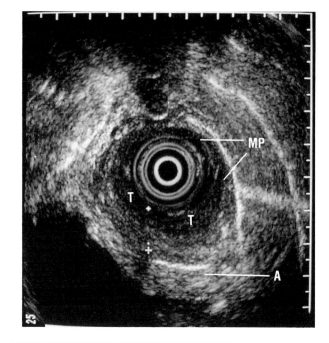

B.

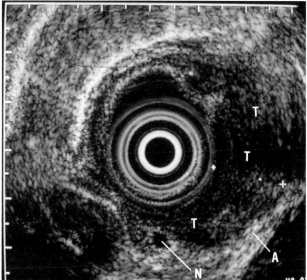

C.

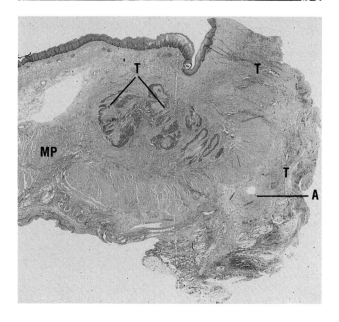

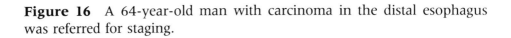

Figure 16 A 64-year-old man with carcinoma in the distal esophagus was referred for staging.

A.
EUS shows a semicircular transmural hypoechoic carcinoma (T) with penetration through the muscularis propria (MP) into the adventitia (A). Note the smaller crystal (CR) of the Aloka nonoptic echoprobe compared with those of the Olympus echoendoscope. AO = aorta, LA = left atrium, V = vertebral body.

B.
CT shows an asymmetric thickening (T) of the esophageal wall. Note the topographic correspondence between EUS and CT. AO = descending aorta, AA = ascending aorta, V = vertebral body, LA = left atrium.

C.
Barium swallow shows a polypoid tumor (T) at the right side.

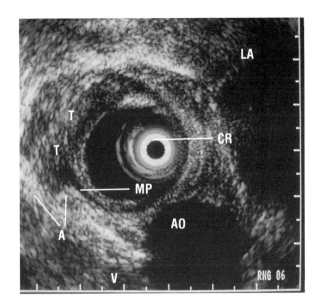

A.

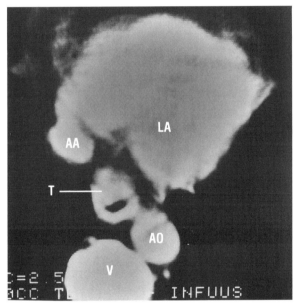

B.

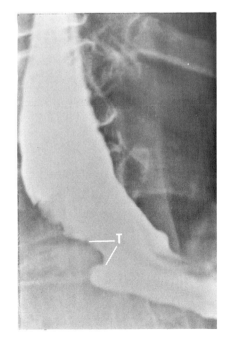

C.

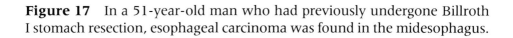

Figure 17 In a 51-year-old man who had previously undergone Billroth I stomach resection, esophageal carcinoma was found in the midesophagus.

A.
EUS shows an intrasubmucosal hypoechoic tumor (T) limited to the submucosa (SM) without penetration into the muscularis propria (MP) located adjacent to the aorta (AO). LA = left atrium.

B.
Another transverse section shows a polypoid hypoechoic tumor (T) with penetration through the muscularis propria (MP) into the adventitia (A). Note the topographic relationship between the aorta (AO) and the carcinoma. LA = left atrium.

C.
Corresponding barium swallow shows a polypoid double contour of the carcinoma (T) localized dorsally. V = vertebral body.

A.

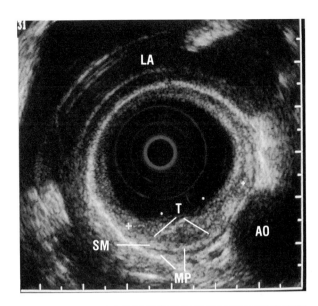

B.

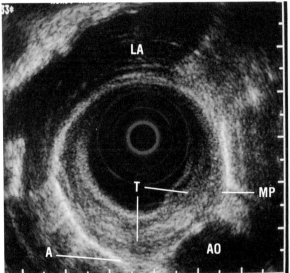

C.

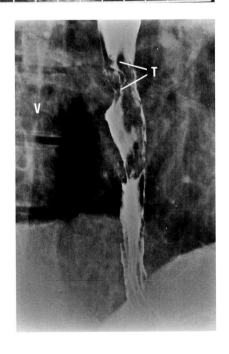

Figure 18 A 59-year-old man with esophageal carcinoma at the middle part of the esophagus found endoscopically was referred for staging.

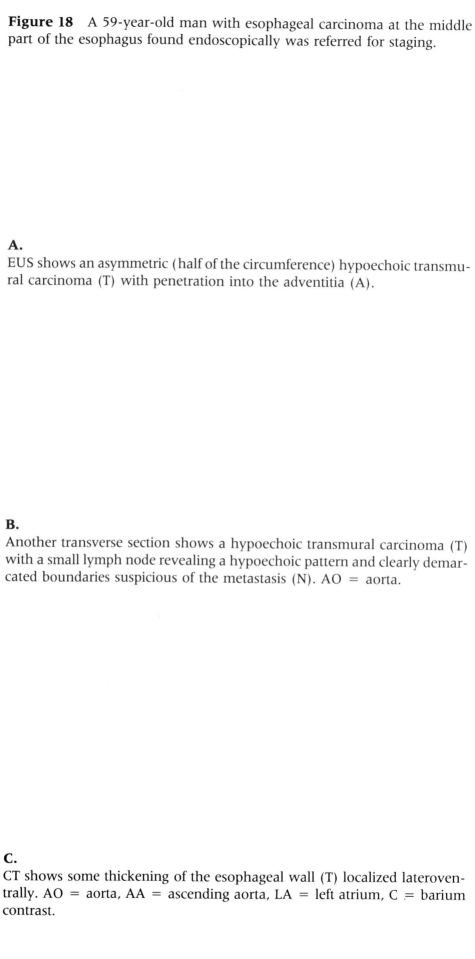

A.
EUS shows an asymmetric (half of the circumference) hypoechoic transmural carcinoma (T) with penetration into the adventitia (A).

B.
Another transverse section shows a hypoechoic transmural carcinoma (T) with a small lymph node revealing a hypoechoic pattern and clearly demarcated boundaries suspicious of the metastasis (N). AO = aorta.

C.
CT shows some thickening of the esophageal wall (T) localized lateroventrally. AO = aorta, AA = ascending aorta, LA = left atrium, C = barium contrast.

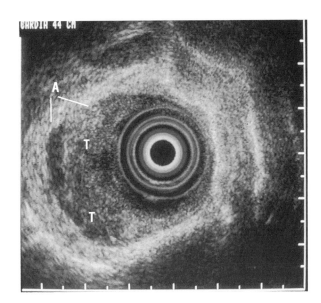

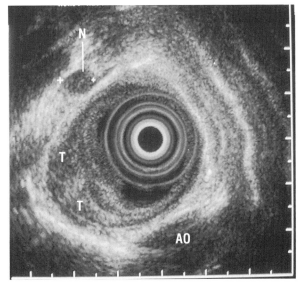

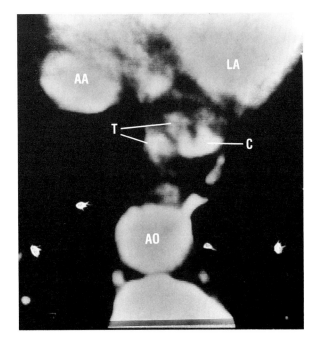

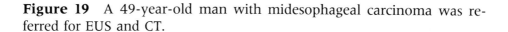

Figure 19 A 49-year-old man with midesophageal carcinoma was referred for EUS and CT.

A.

EUS shows an ulcerative (U) carcinoma (T) with some nodular margins penetrating through the muscularis propria (MP) into the adventitia (A). Note a small lymph node with hypoechoic pattern and clearly demarcated boundaries suspicious of metastasis (N). AV = azygos vein, AO = aorta, LA = left atrium, V = vertebral body.

B.

Corresponding CT shows a polypoid thickening of the esophageal wall (T) adjacent to the left atrium (LA). AV = azygos vein, AO = aorta, V = vertebra.

C.

Barium swallow shows an ulcerative (U) carcinoma with some nodular margins (arrows).

A.

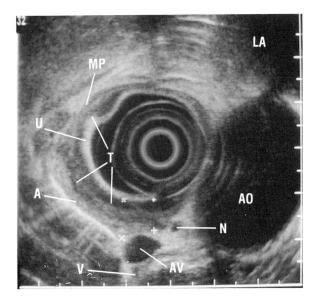

B.

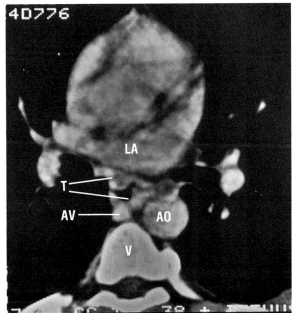

C.

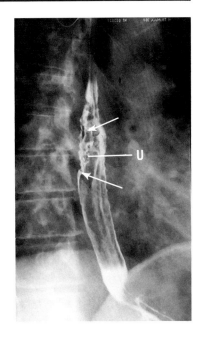

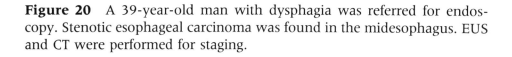

Figure 20 A 39-year-old man with dysphagia was referred for endoscopy. Stenotic esophageal carcinoma was found in the midesophagus. EUS and CT were performed for staging.

A.
EUS shows a semicircular (three-fourths of the circumference) hypoechoic tumor (T) with penetration (arrows) into the azygos vein (AV) directly adjacent to the vertebra (V). Note the aortic arch (AR) at the contralateral side of the azygos vein. TR = trachea, SVC = superior vena cava.

B.
Corresponding CT shows some circular thickening of the esophageal wall (T) between the azygos vein (AV) and aortic arch (AR). TR = trachea, SVC = superior vena cava.

C.
Barium swallow shows a stenotic carcinoma (T) in the middle part of the esophagus.

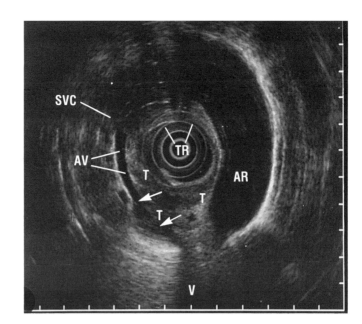

A.

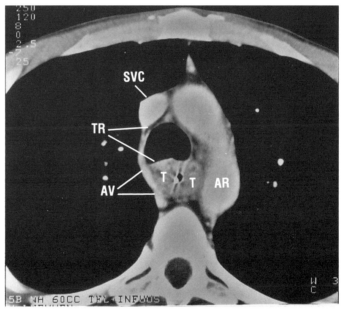

B.

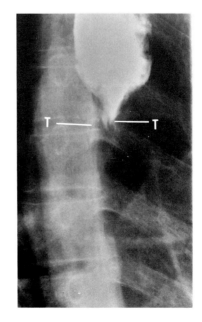

C.

Figure 21 A 65-year-old man with a stenotic esophageal carcinoma was admitted to the hospital. A feeding tube was inserted because of his poor nutritional condition. EUS and CT were performed for staging.

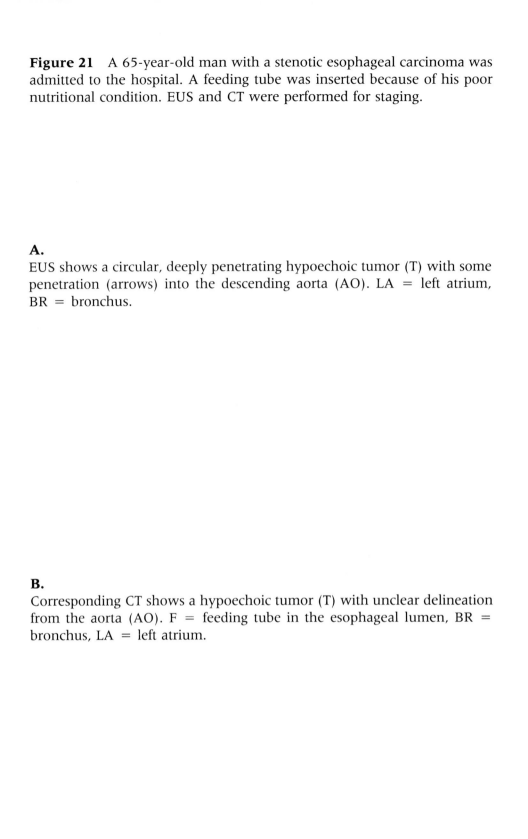

A.
EUS shows a circular, deeply penetrating hypoechoic tumor (T) with some penetration (arrows) into the descending aorta (AO). LA = left atrium, BR = bronchus.

B.
Corresponding CT shows a hypoechoic tumor (T) with unclear delineation from the aorta (AO). F = feeding tube in the esophageal lumen, BR = bronchus, LA = left atrium.

C.
Endoscopy shows a polypoid esophageal carcinoma (arrows).

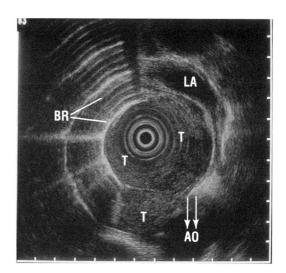

A.

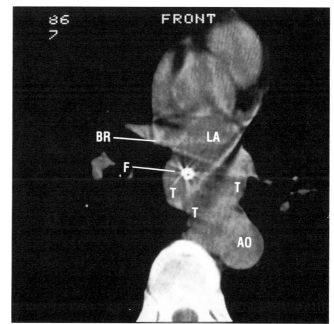

B.

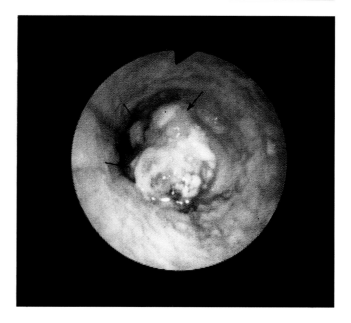

C.

Figure 22 A 64-year-old woman with a small malignant gastric ulcer suspicious of early gastric carcinoma found endoscopically was referred for preoperative staging.

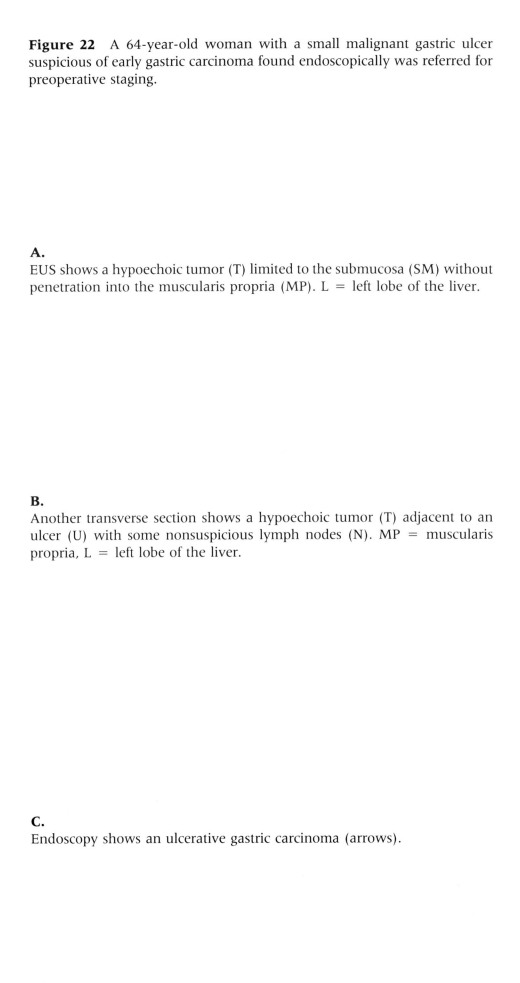

A.
EUS shows a hypoechoic tumor (T) limited to the submucosa (SM) without penetration into the muscularis propria (MP). L = left lobe of the liver.

B.
Another transverse section shows a hypoechoic tumor (T) adjacent to an ulcer (U) with some nonsuspicious lymph nodes (N). MP = muscularis propria, L = left lobe of the liver.

C.
Endoscopy shows an ulcerative gastric carcinoma (arrows).

A.

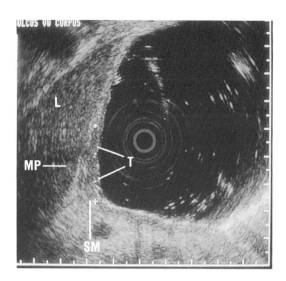

B.

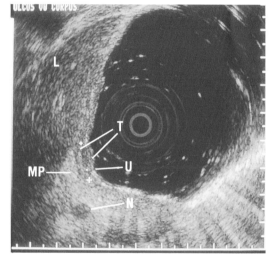

C.

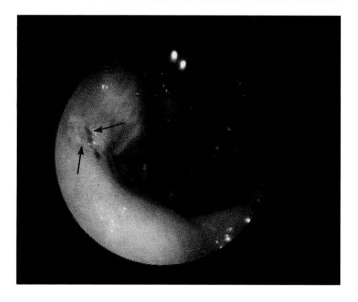

Figure 23 In a 60-year-old man, a small malignant ulcer was found endoscopically at the anastomosis after Billroth I gastrectomy. He had been treated 38 years earlier for a peptic ulcer.

A.
EUS shows a hypoechoic tumor (T) limited to the mucosa adjacent to an ulcer (U). Note the relatively superficial infiltration bordering the hyperechoic submucosa (SM). L = left lobe of the liver, MP = muscularis propria.

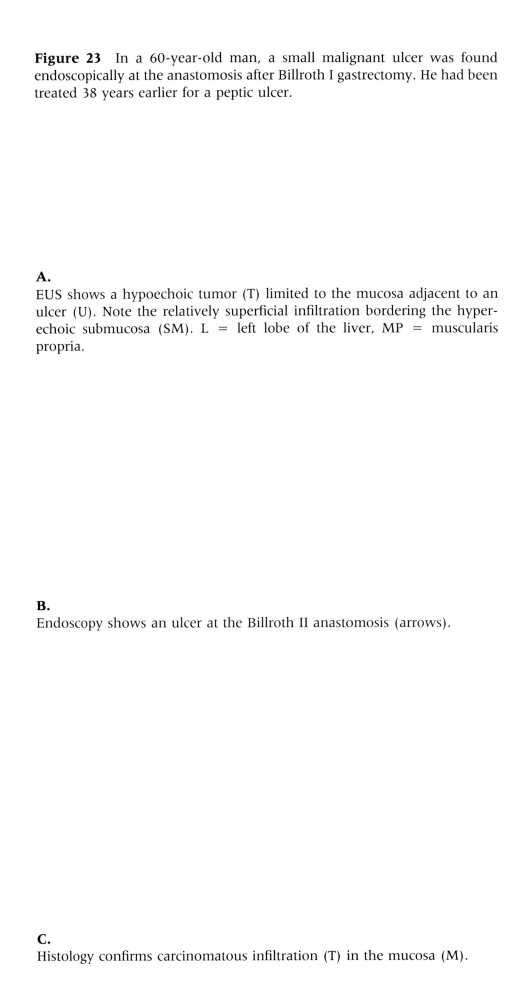

B.
Endoscopy shows an ulcer at the Billroth II anastomosis (arrows).

C.
Histology confirms carcinomatous infiltration (T) in the mucosa (M).

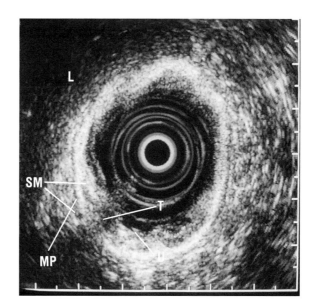

A.

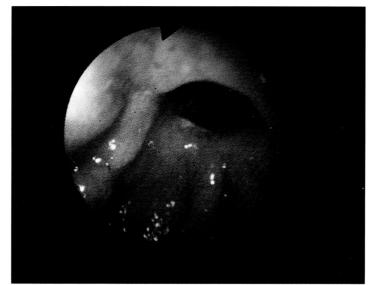

B.

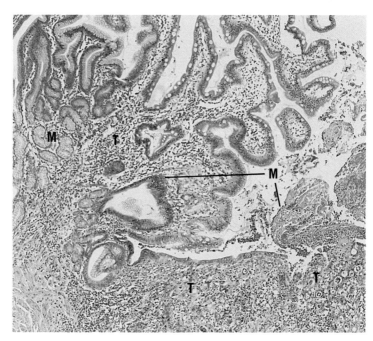

C.

Figure 24 An 81-year-old woman with an extensive villous adenoma in the body of the stomach found endoscopically was referred for staging.

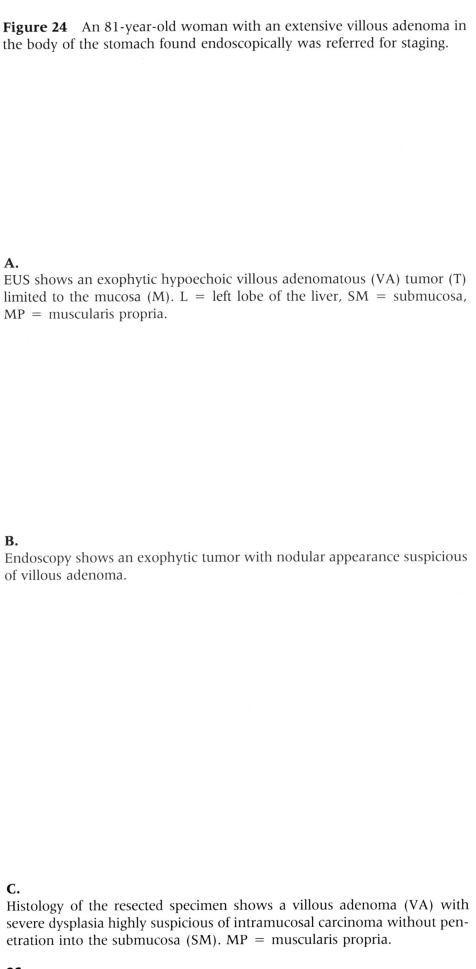

A.
EUS shows an exophytic hypoechoic villous adenomatous (VA) tumor (T) limited to the mucosa (M). L = left lobe of the liver, SM = submucosa, MP = muscularis propria.

B.
Endoscopy shows an exophytic tumor with nodular appearance suspicious of villous adenoma.

C.
Histology of the resected specimen shows a villous adenoma (VA) with severe dysplasia highly suspicious of intramucosal carcinoma without penetration into the submucosa (SM). MP = muscularis propria.

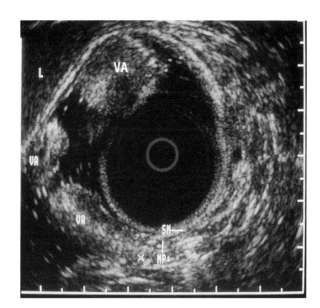

A.

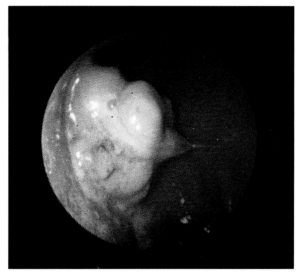

B.

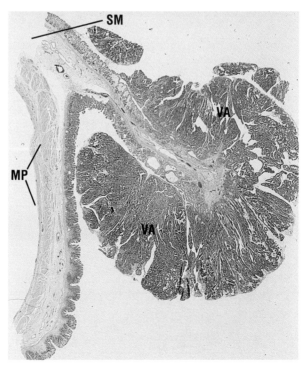

C.

Figure 25 A 68-year-old man with a carcinoma in the body of the stomach was referred for preoperative staging.

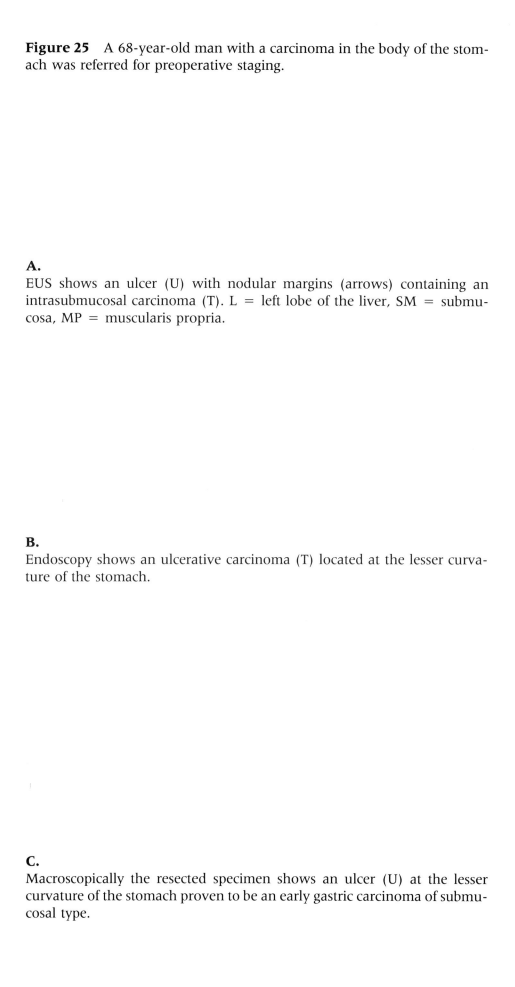

A.
EUS shows an ulcer (U) with nodular margins (arrows) containing an intrasubmucosal carcinoma (T). L = left lobe of the liver, SM = submucosa, MP = muscularis propria.

B.
Endoscopy shows an ulcerative carcinoma (T) located at the lesser curvature of the stomach.

C.
Macroscopically the resected specimen shows an ulcer (U) at the lesser curvature of the stomach proven to be an early gastric carcinoma of submucosal type.

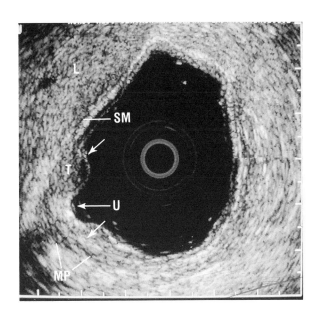

A.

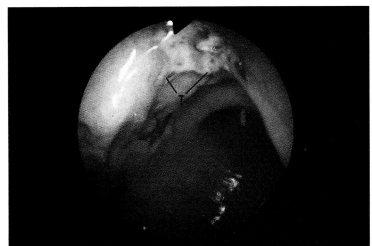

B.

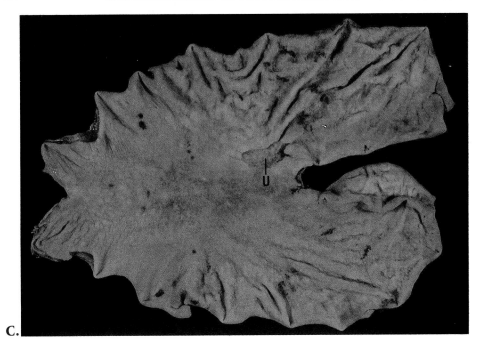

C.

Figure 26 A 79-year-old man with recurrent abdominal pain was referred for gastroscopy. A malignant ulcer was found at the junction between the fundus and body of the stomach.

A.
EUS shows a hypoechoic intrasubmucosal carcinoma (T) adjacent to an ulcer (U).

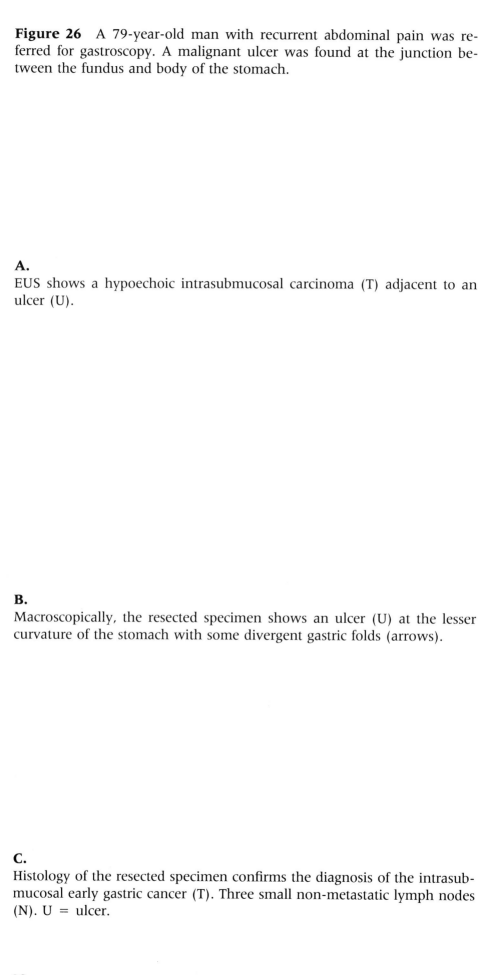

B.
Macroscopically, the resected specimen shows an ulcer (U) at the lesser curvature of the stomach with some divergent gastric folds (arrows).

C.
Histology of the resected specimen confirms the diagnosis of the intrasubmucosal early gastric cancer (T). Three small non-metastatic lymph nodes (N). U = ulcer.

A.

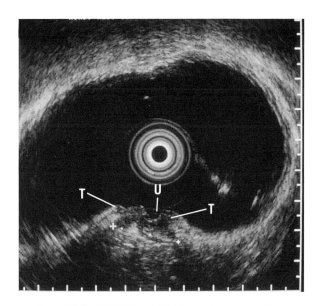

B.

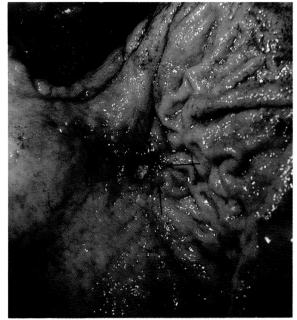

C.

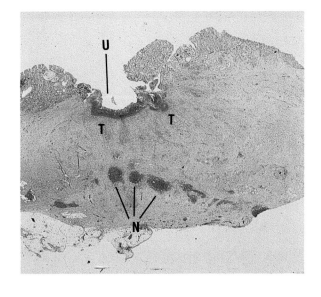

Figure 27 A 57-year-old man with gastric carcinoma at the lesser curvature of corpus was referred for staging to assess resectability.

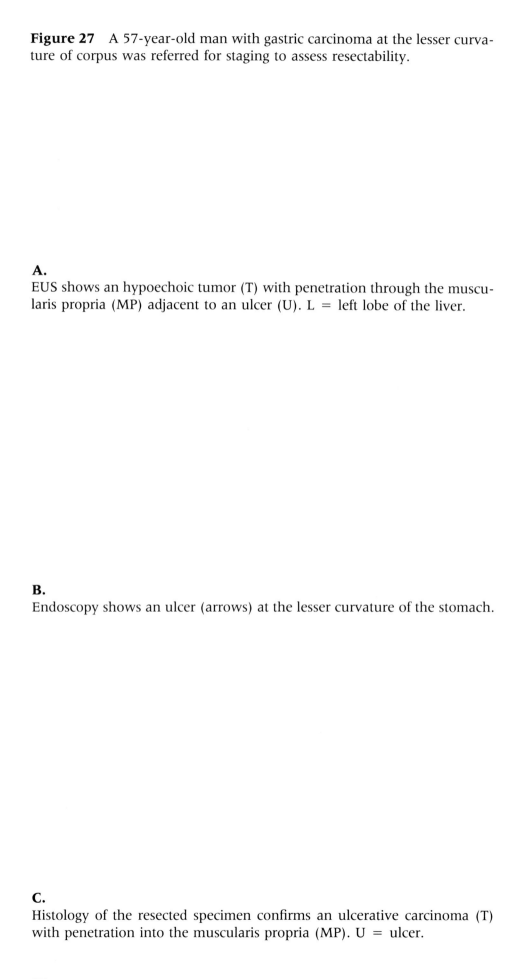

A.
EUS shows an hypoechoic tumor (T) with penetration through the muscularis propria (MP) adjacent to an ulcer (U). L = left lobe of the liver.

B.
Endoscopy shows an ulcer (arrows) at the lesser curvature of the stomach.

C.
Histology of the resected specimen confirms an ulcerative carcinoma (T) with penetration into the muscularis propria (MP). U = ulcer.

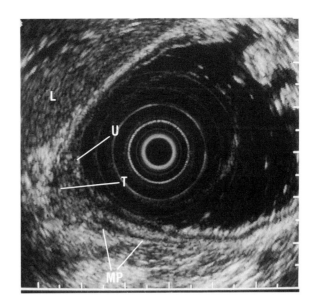

A.

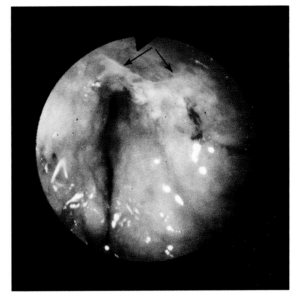

B.

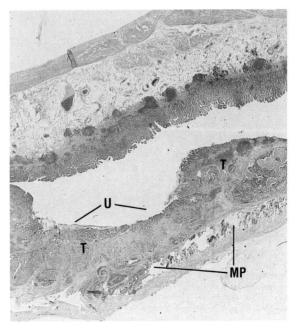

C.

Figure 28 A 37-year-old woman with recurrent gastric ulcer was referred for endoscopy. Multiple biopsies ascertained the diagnosis of signet-ring cell carcinoma.

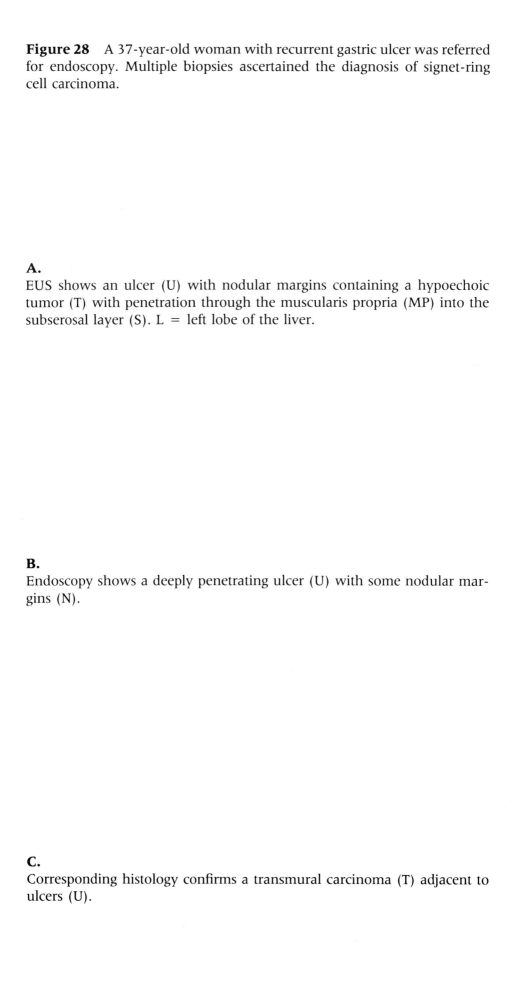

A.
EUS shows an ulcer (U) with nodular margins containing a hypoechoic tumor (T) with penetration through the muscularis propria (MP) into the subserosal layer (S). L = left lobe of the liver.

B.
Endoscopy shows a deeply penetrating ulcer (U) with some nodular margins (N).

C.
Corresponding histology confirms a transmural carcinoma (T) adjacent to ulcers (U).

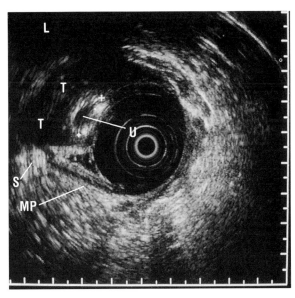

A.

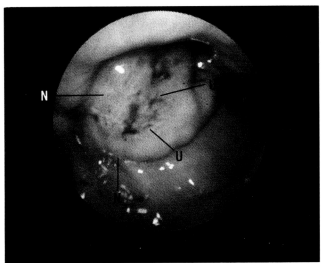

B.

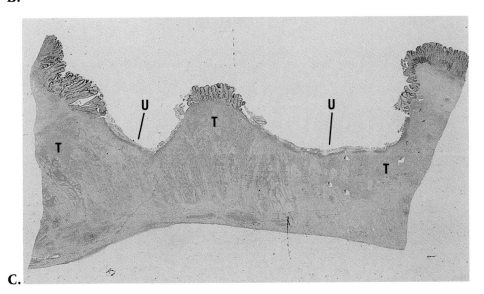

C.

Figure 29 A 67-year-old man with malignant gastric ulcer was referred for preoperative staging.

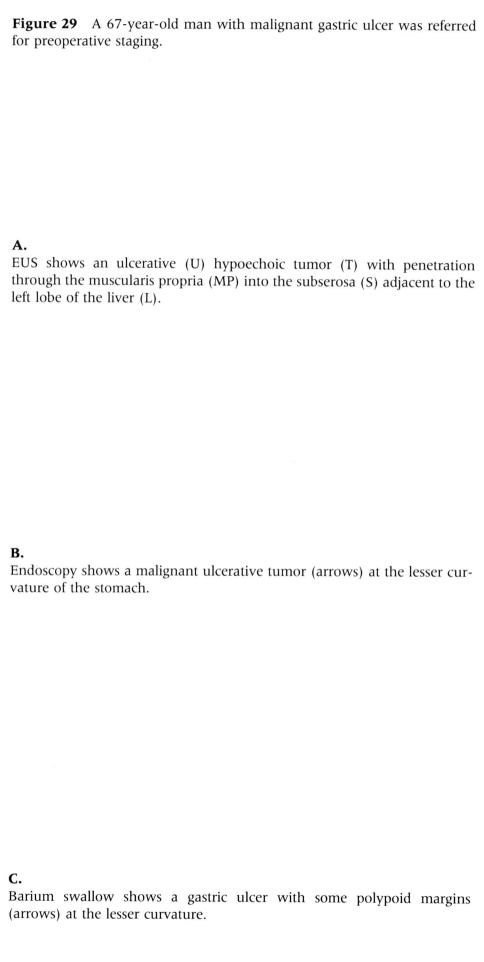

A.
EUS shows an ulcerative (U) hypoechoic tumor (T) with penetration through the muscularis propria (MP) into the subserosa (S) adjacent to the left lobe of the liver (L).

B.
Endoscopy shows a malignant ulcerative tumor (arrows) at the lesser curvature of the stomach.

C.
Barium swallow shows a gastric ulcer with some polypoid margins (arrows) at the lesser curvature.

A.

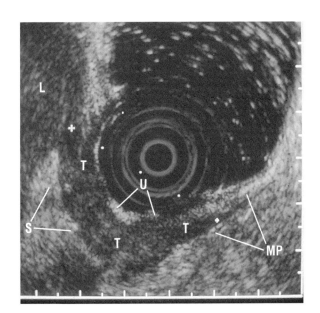

B.

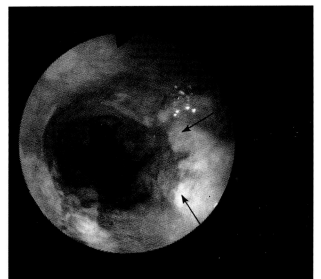

C.

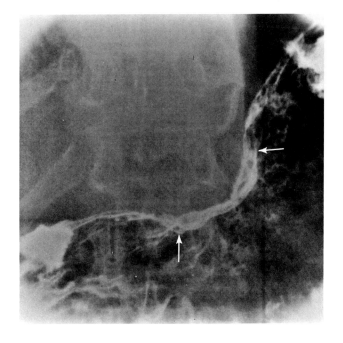

Figure 30 A 64-year-old man with polypoid carcinoma found endoscopically was referred for preoperative staging.

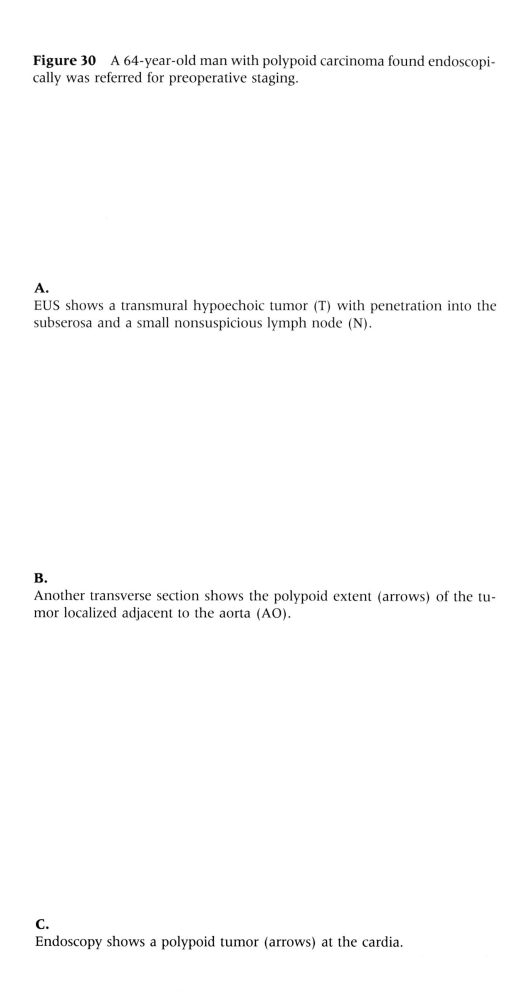

A.
EUS shows a transmural hypoechoic tumor (T) with penetration into the subserosa and a small nonsuspicious lymph node (N).

B.
Another transverse section shows the polypoid extent (arrows) of the tumor localized adjacent to the aorta (AO).

C.
Endoscopy shows a polypoid tumor (arrows) at the cardia.

A.

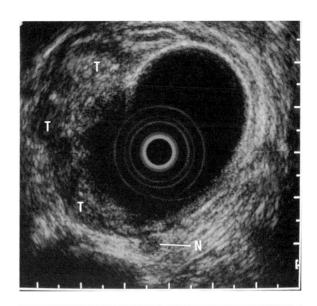

B.

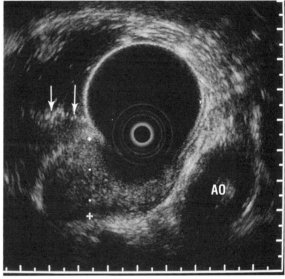

C.

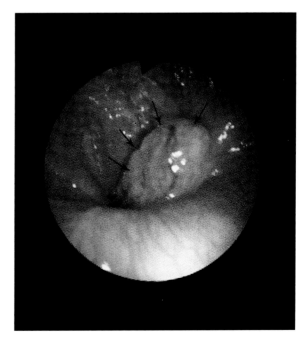

Figure 31 A 75-year-old man with dysphagia was referred for endoscopy. Diffuse submucosal tumor infiltration strongly suspicious of linitis plastica was found.

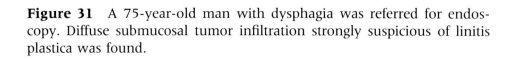

A.
EUS shows a diffuse intrasubmucosal carcinoma (T) with minimal penetration (arrows) into the muscularis propria (MP). Note the thickening of the muscularis propria, presumably due to hypertrophy secondary to diffuse carcinomatous infiltration (linitis plastica).

B.
CT shows some thickening (T) of the gastric wall without further detailed information because the muscularis propria cannot be imaged.

C.
Histology of the resected specimen confirms diffuse submucosal carcinomatous infiltration (T) with some penetration (arrows) into the muscularis propria (MP).

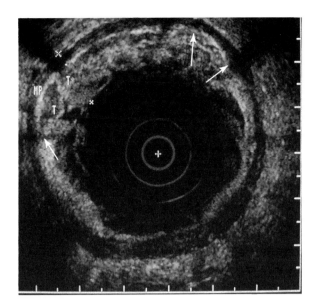

A.

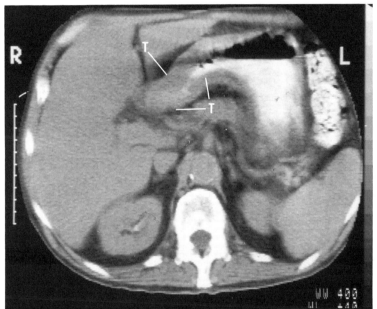

B.

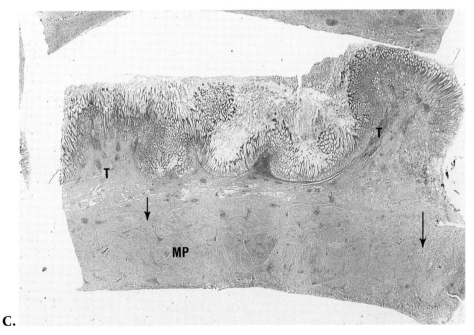

C.

101

Figure 32 A 60-year-old man with diffuse double contours in the stomach strongly suspicious of linitis plastica, found radiographically, was referred for preoperative staging.

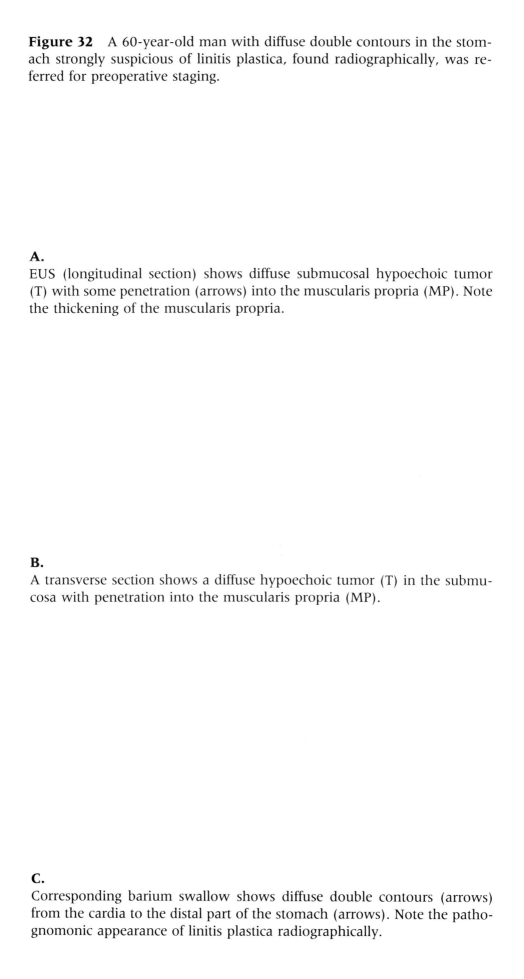

A.
EUS (longitudinal section) shows diffuse submucosal hypoechoic tumor (T) with some penetration (arrows) into the muscularis propria (MP). Note the thickening of the muscularis propria.

B.
A transverse section shows a diffuse hypoechoic tumor (T) in the submucosa with penetration into the muscularis propria (MP).

C.
Corresponding barium swallow shows diffuse double contours (arrows) from the cardia to the distal part of the stomach (arrows). Note the pathognomonic appearance of linitis plastica radiographically.

A.

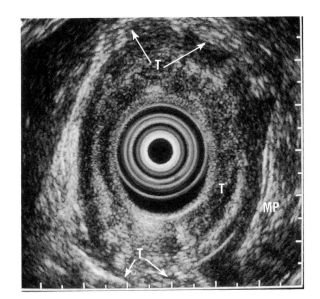

B.

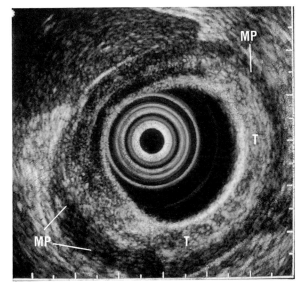

C.

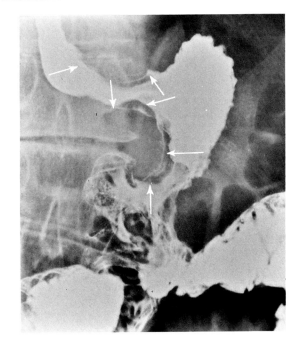

Figure 33 A 70-year-old man with dysphagia was referred for endoscopy. A cardia carcinoma was found endoscopically. Preoperative staging was performed for assessment of resectability.

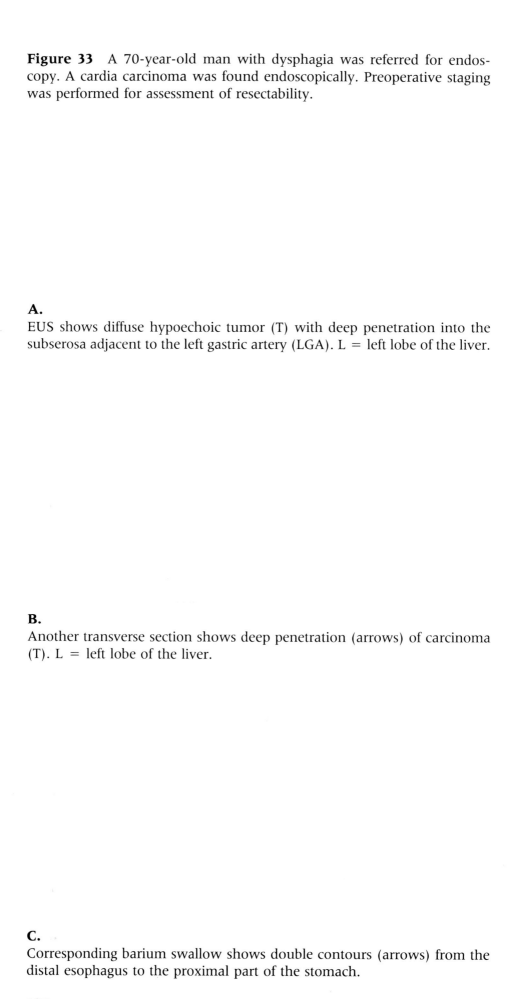

A.
EUS shows diffuse hypoechoic tumor (T) with deep penetration into the subserosa adjacent to the left gastric artery (LGA). L = left lobe of the liver.

B.
Another transverse section shows deep penetration (arrows) of carcinoma (T). L = left lobe of the liver.

C.
Corresponding barium swallow shows double contours (arrows) from the distal esophagus to the proximal part of the stomach.

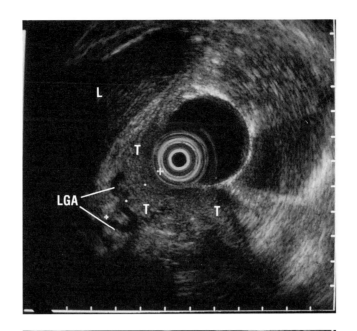

A.

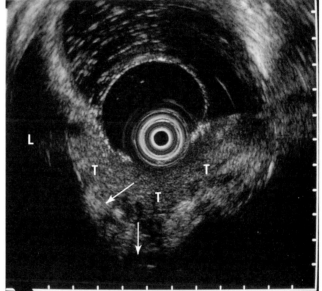

B.

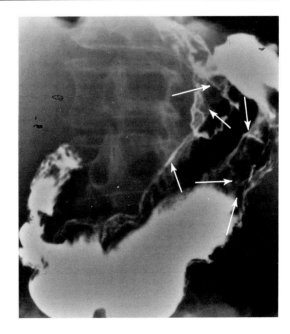

C.

Figure 34 A 75-year-old man with gastric carcinoma was referred for staging.

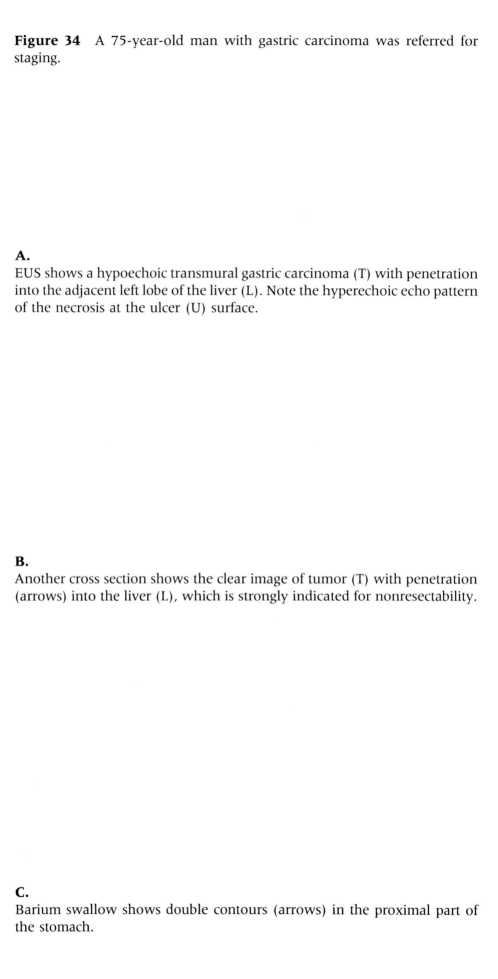

A.
EUS shows a hypoechoic transmural gastric carcinoma (T) with penetration into the adjacent left lobe of the liver (L). Note the hyperechoic echo pattern of the necrosis at the ulcer (U) surface.

B.
Another cross section shows the clear image of tumor (T) with penetration (arrows) into the liver (L), which is strongly indicated for nonresectability.

C.
Barium swallow shows double contours (arrows) in the proximal part of the stomach.

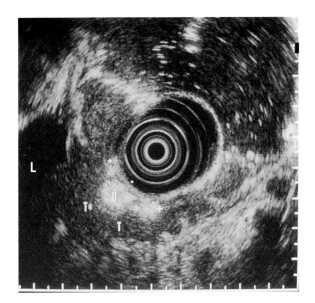

A.

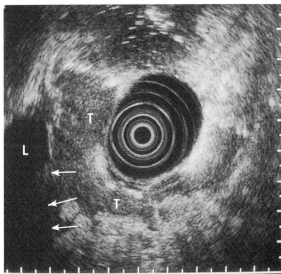

B.

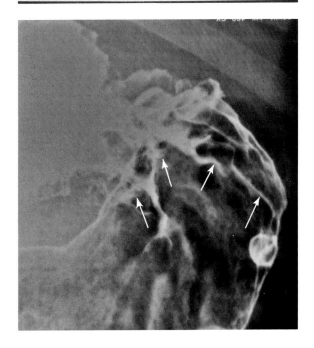

C.

Figure 35 A 40-year-old man with a primary duodenal carcinoma found endoscopically was referred for staging.

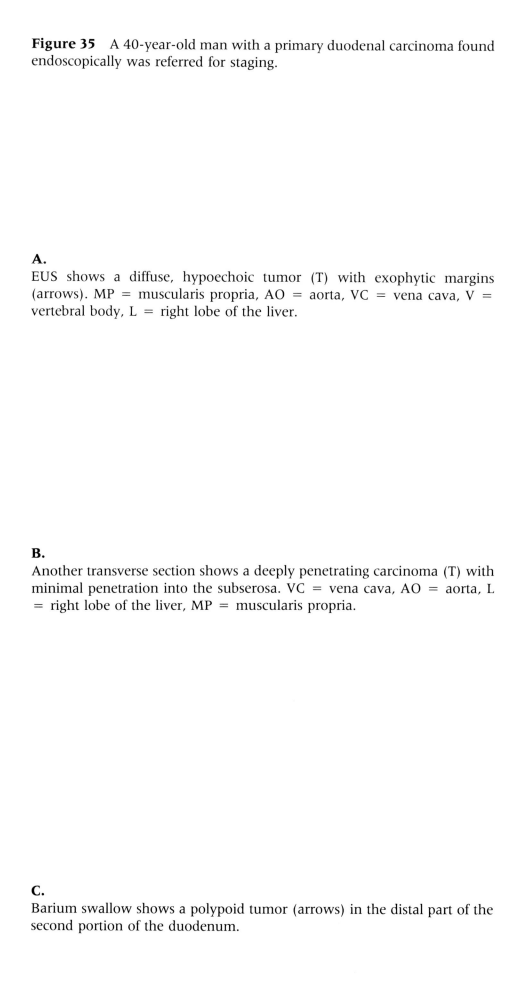

A.
EUS shows a diffuse, hypoechoic tumor (T) with exophytic margins (arrows). MP = muscularis propria, AO = aorta, VC = vena cava, V = vertebral body, L = right lobe of the liver.

B.
Another transverse section shows a deeply penetrating carcinoma (T) with minimal penetration into the subserosa. VC = vena cava, AO = aorta, L = right lobe of the liver, MP = muscularis propria.

C.
Barium swallow shows a polypoid tumor (arrows) in the distal part of the second portion of the duodenum.

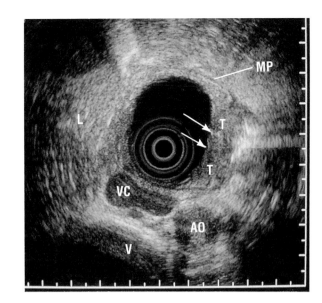

A.

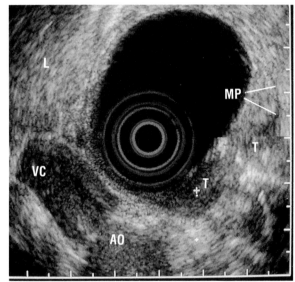

B.

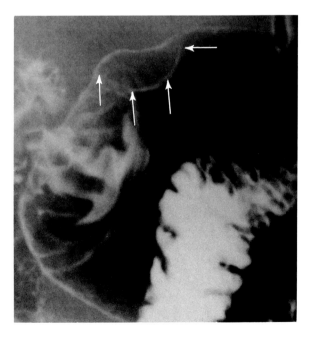

C.

Figure 36 A 48-year-old woman with painless jaundice was referred for ERCP. Ampullary carcinoma with dilation of the common bile duct directly adjacent to the papilla of Vater was found.

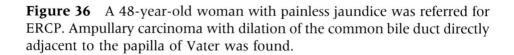

A.
EUS shows a transmural duodenal carcinoma (T) with penetration of the subserosal layer (S) localized dorsally adjacent to the aorta (AO). P = pancreas, V = vertebral body, VC = vena cava, L = liver.

B.
Another cross section shows a transmural tumor (T) with penetration through the muscularis propria (MP) into the subserosa. Note the close proximity of the tumor to the pancreas (P). L= right lobe of the liver, AO = aorta.

C.
Corresponding histology shows a polypoid carcinoma (T) with some penetration through the muscularis propria (MP) into the subserosal layer (S) with no evidence of penetration into the pancreas (P).

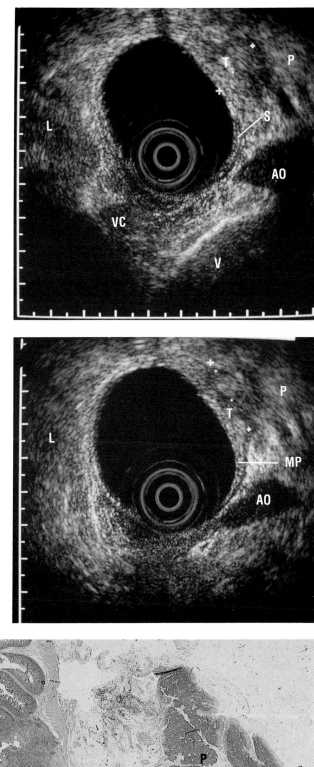

A.

B.

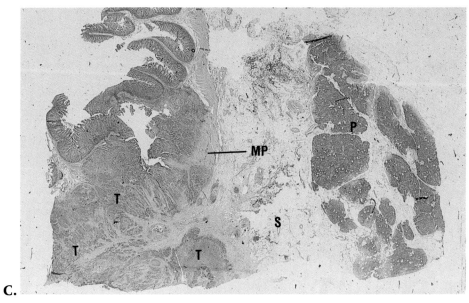

C.

Figure 37 A 50-year-old man was referred for abdominal sonography for the evaluation of gallstone disease. Dilation of the extrahepatic bile duct was found. ERCP revealed a pedunculated ampullary ulcerative carcinoma without successful filling of the common bile duct and pancreatic duct. EUS was performed for preoperative staging.

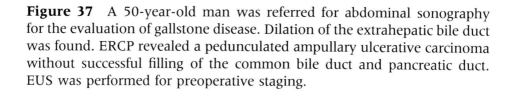

A.
EUS shows dilatation of the common bile duct (CBD) and pancreatic duct (PD) directly adjacent to the ampulla of Vater with a common channel in the ampulla of Vater (A).

B.
Another transverse section of a pedunculated tumor shows a hypoechoic tumor (T) penetrated into the deeper layer of the mucosa with a central ulcer (U) consistent with an intramucosal cancer.

C.
Corresponding histology confirms an ampullary carcinoma (T) penetrating into the muscularis mucosae (MM) of the pedunculated ampulla.

A.

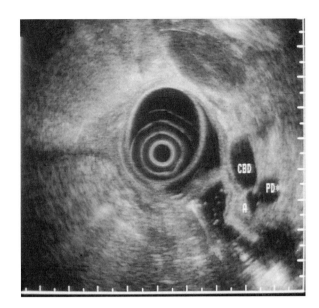

B.

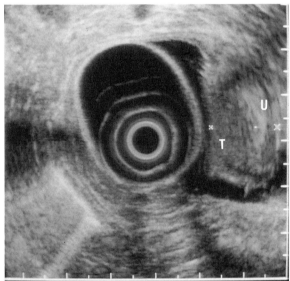

C.

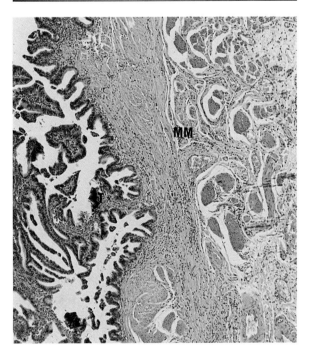

Figure 38 A 65-year-old woman with obstructive jaundice and malaise was referred for ERCP. Endoscopic biopsy ascertained the diagnosis of ampullary carcinoma.

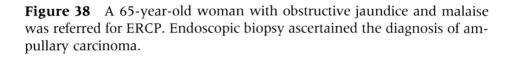

A.
EUS shows a hypoechoic tumor (T) in the ampulla of Vater with penetration into the muscularis propria (MP) but with no evidence of penetration into the pancreas (P). L = right lobe of the liver.

B.
EUS of the resected specimen shows an ampullary carcinoma (T) with penetration into the muscularis propria (MP). Note the hyperechoic pattern (arrows) representing a tumor-free zone between the tumor (T) and pancreas (P).

C.
Corresponding histology confirms a polypoid ampullary carcinoma (T) with penetration into the muscularis propria (MP). Note the tumor-free (arrows) subserosal layer between the pancreas (P) and the tumor.

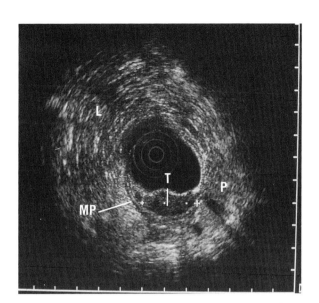

A.

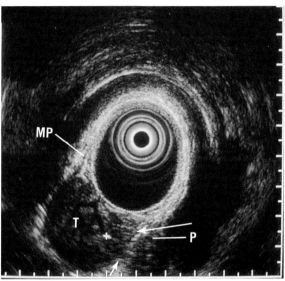

B.

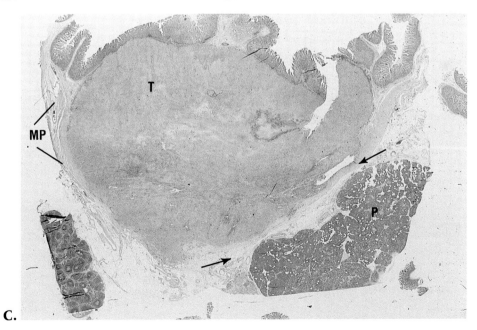

C.

115

Figure 39 Same patient as Figure 38.

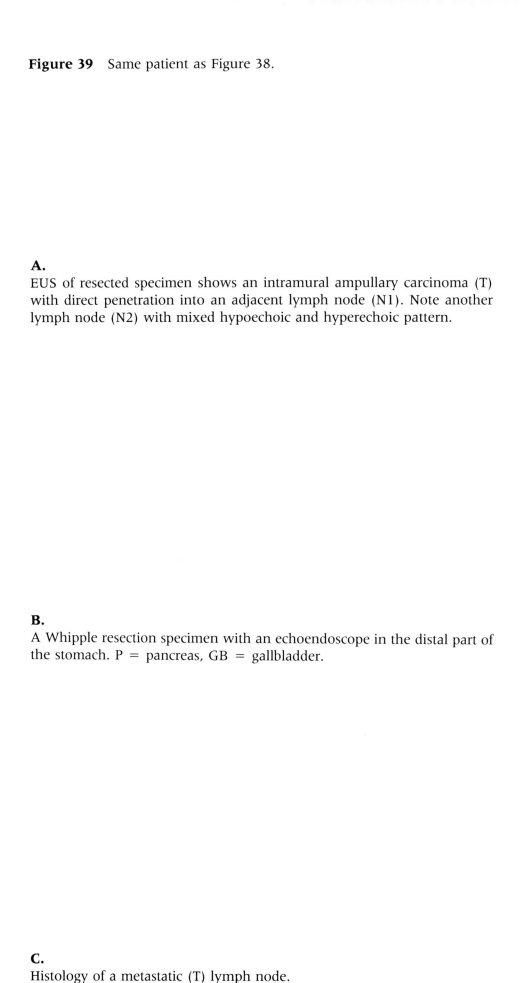

A.
EUS of resected specimen shows an intramural ampullary carcinoma (T) with direct penetration into an adjacent lymph node (N1). Note another lymph node (N2) with mixed hypoechoic and hyperechoic pattern.

B.
A Whipple resection specimen with an echoendoscope in the distal part of the stomach. P = pancreas, GB = gallbladder.

C.
Histology of a metastatic (T) lymph node.

116

A.

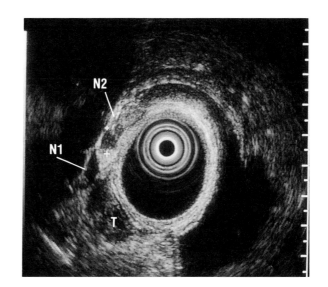

B.

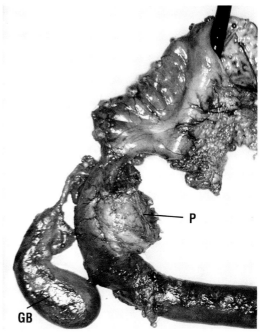

C.

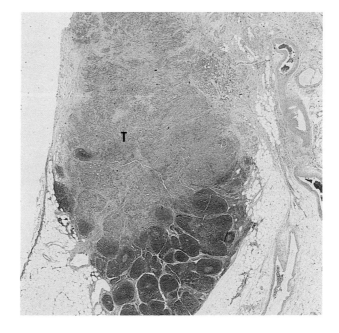

Figure 40 In a 61-year-old man ERCP and EUS were performed because of obstructive jaundice. The endoscopic biopsy of the ampulla of Vater ascertained the diagnosis of carcinoma.

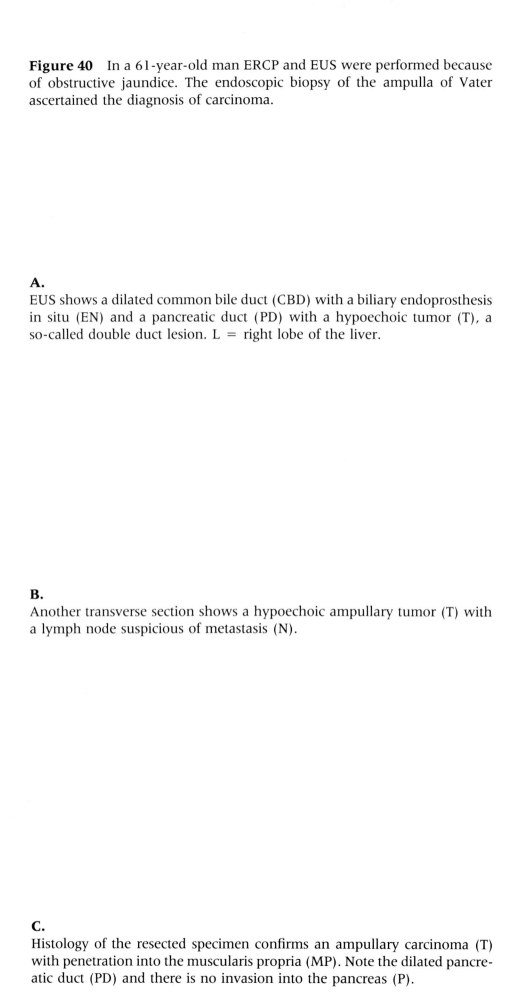

A.
EUS shows a dilated common bile duct (CBD) with a biliary endoprosthesis in situ (EN) and a pancreatic duct (PD) with a hypoechoic tumor (T), a so-called double duct lesion. L = right lobe of the liver.

B.
Another transverse section shows a hypoechoic ampullary tumor (T) with a lymph node suspicious of metastasis (N).

C.
Histology of the resected specimen confirms an ampullary carcinoma (T) with penetration into the muscularis propria (MP). Note the dilated pancreatic duct (PD) and there is no invasion into the pancreas (P).

A.

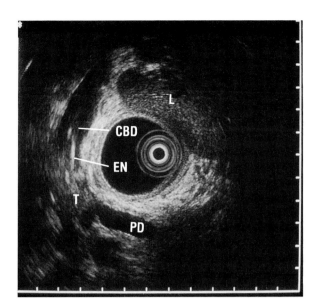

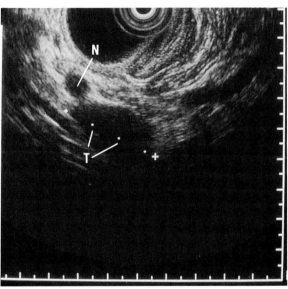

B.

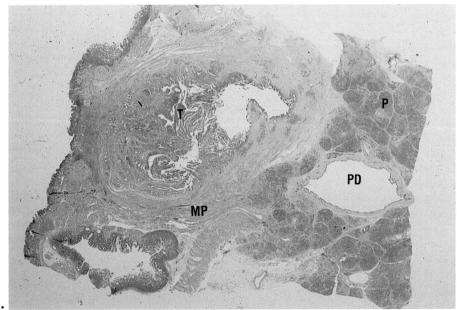

C.

119

Figure 41 A 70-year-old woman was referred for EUS because of ampullary carcinoma found at ERCP.

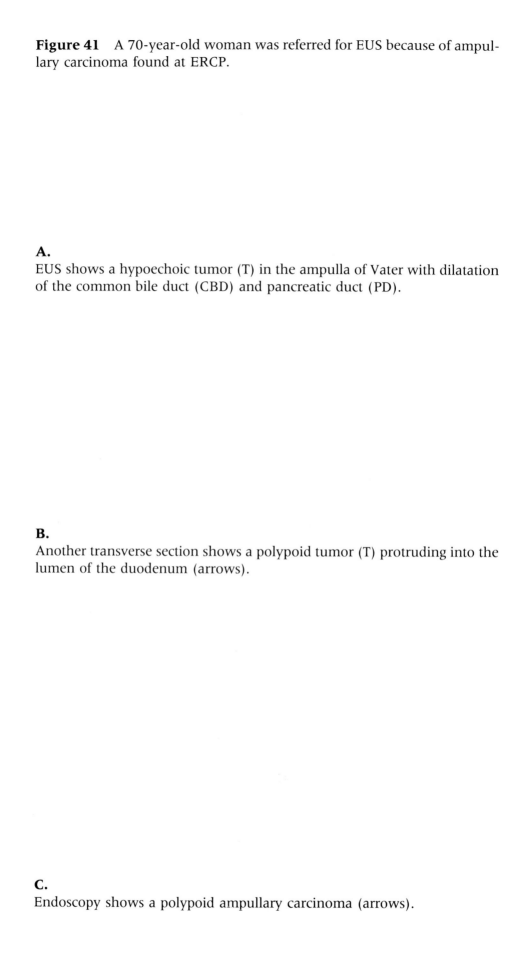

A.
EUS shows a hypoechoic tumor (T) in the ampulla of Vater with dilatation of the common bile duct (CBD) and pancreatic duct (PD).

B.
Another transverse section shows a polypoid tumor (T) protruding into the lumen of the duodenum (arrows).

C.
Endoscopy shows a polypoid ampullary carcinoma (arrows).

A.

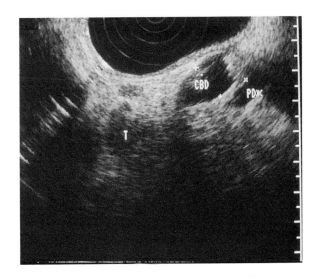

B.

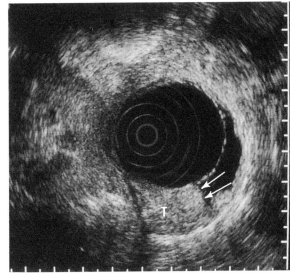

C.

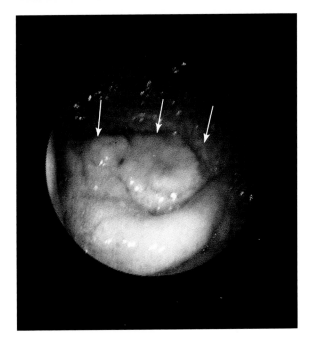

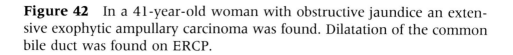

Figure 42 In a 41-year-old woman with obstructive jaundice an extensive exophytic ampullary carcinoma was found. Dilatation of the common bile duct was found on ERCP.

A.
EUS shows a hypoechoic tumor (T) with penetration into the dilated common bile duct (CBD) and some penetration into the pancreatic parenchyma with a nondilated pancreatic duct (PD). P = pancreas.

B.
Another transverse section shows a hypoechoic tumor (T) penetrating through the muscularis propria (MP) into the adjacent pancreas (P).

C.
Histology of the resected specimen confirms an ampullary carcinoma (T) with penetration through the muscularis propria (MP) into (arrows) the pancreas (P).

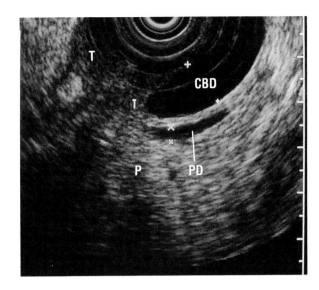

A.

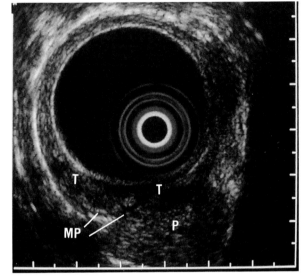

B.

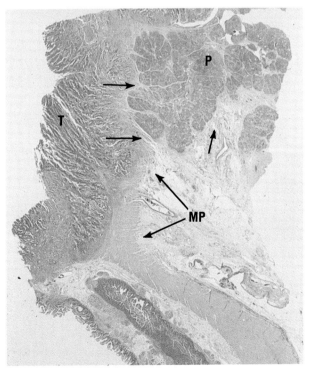

C.

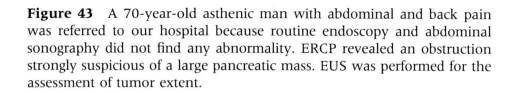

Figure 43 A 70-year-old asthenic man with abdominal and back pain was referred to our hospital because routine endoscopy and abdominal sonography did not find any abnormality. ERCP revealed an obstruction strongly suspicious of a large pancreatic mass. EUS was performed for the assessment of tumor extent.

A.
EUS shows an intraductal pancreatic carcinoma (T) within a dilated pancreatic duct (PD). SV = splenic vein, P = pancreas.

B.
Another transverse section shows an intraductal tumor (T) with some penetration (arrows) into the adjacent pancreas (P) with a diameter less than 20 mm (T1).

C.
Corresponding histology of the resected specimen shows epithelial dysplasia (EP) with carcinomatous infiltration (T) surrounding the dilated pancreatic duct (PD).

A.

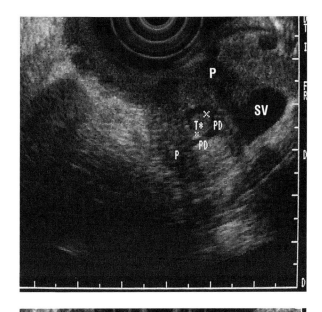

B.

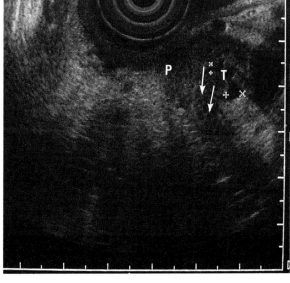

C.

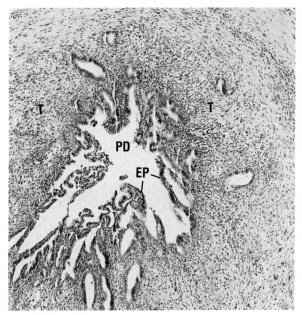

Figure 44 In a 51-year-old man, a biliary endoprosthesis was inserted because of obstructive jaundice. Preoperative EUS was performed for staging.

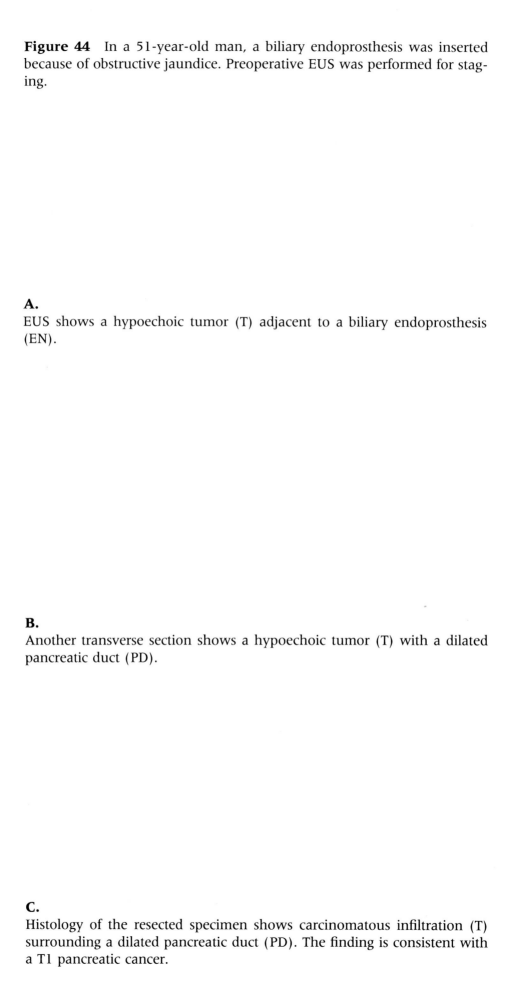

A.
EUS shows a hypoechoic tumor (T) adjacent to a biliary endoprosthesis (EN).

B.
Another transverse section shows a hypoechoic tumor (T) with a dilated pancreatic duct (PD).

C.
Histology of the resected specimen shows carcinomatous infiltration (T) surrounding a dilated pancreatic duct (PD). The finding is consistent with a T1 pancreatic cancer.

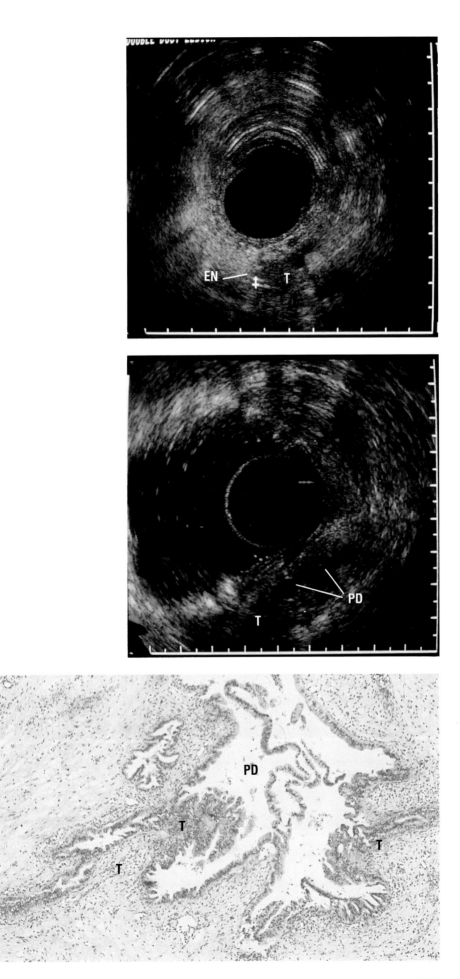

A.

B.

C.

127

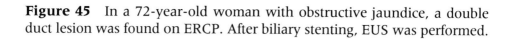

Figure 45 In a 72-year-old woman with obstructive jaundice, a double duct lesion was found on ERCP. After biliary stenting, EUS was performed.

A.

EUS shows a hypoechoic tumor (T) with penetration into the adjacent peripancreatic tissue (arrows). GB = gallbladder with aerobili (AE). P = pancreas.

B.

Another transverse section shows a hypoechoic pancreatic carcinoma (T) with penetration (arrows) into the peripancreatic tissue and common bile duct (CBD) with an endoprosthesis (EN). PD = pancreatic duct.

C.

Histology confirms a pancreatic cancer (T) with peripancreatic infiltration and dilated pancreatic duct (PD) consistent with a T2 carcinoma.

A.

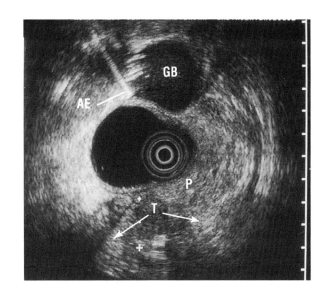

B.

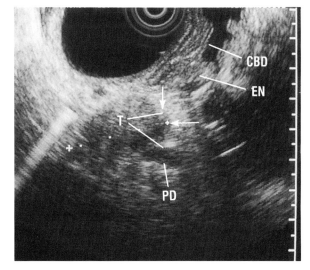

C.

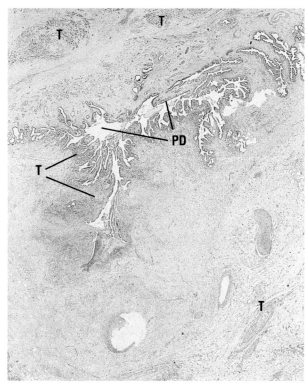

129

Figure 46 A 72-year-old man was referred for EUS because of weight loss, abdominal discomfort, and cholestiasis.

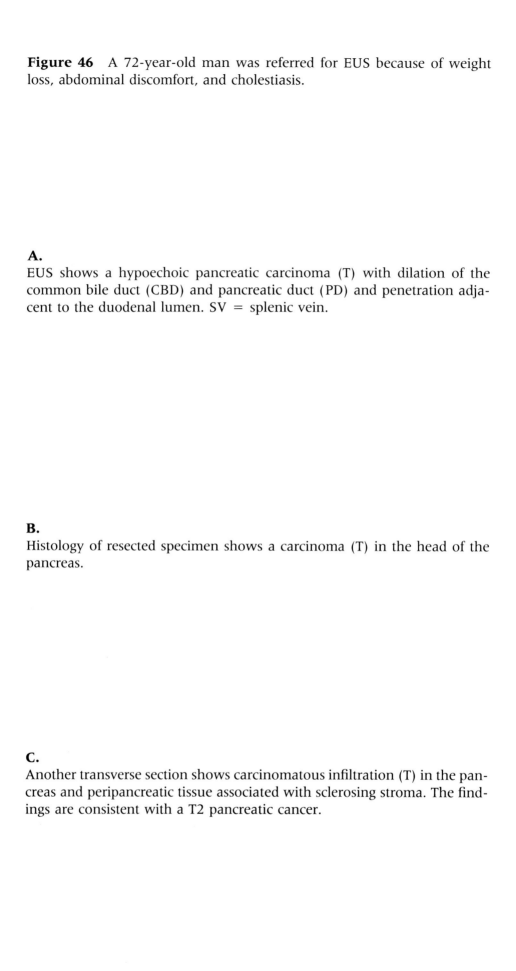

A.
EUS shows a hypoechoic pancreatic carcinoma (T) with dilation of the common bile duct (CBD) and pancreatic duct (PD) and penetration adjacent to the duodenal lumen. SV = splenic vein.

B.
Histology of resected specimen shows a carcinoma (T) in the head of the pancreas.

C.
Another transverse section shows carcinomatous infiltration (T) in the pancreas and peripancreatic tissue associated with sclerosing stroma. The findings are consistent with a T2 pancreatic cancer.

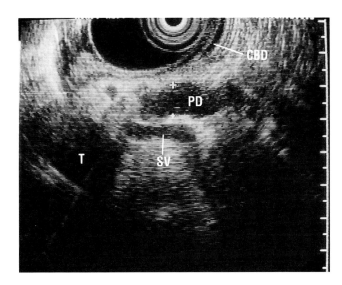

A.

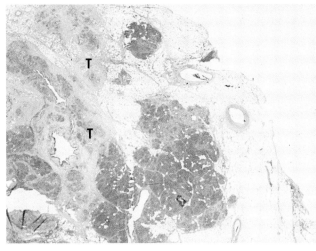

B.

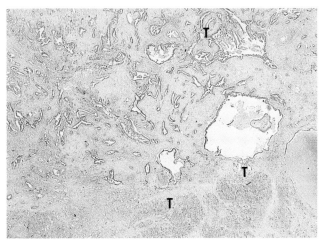

C.

131

Figure 47   A 45-year-old man with obstructive jaundice was referred for staging. A biliary endoprosthesis was inserted for decompression prior to EUS.

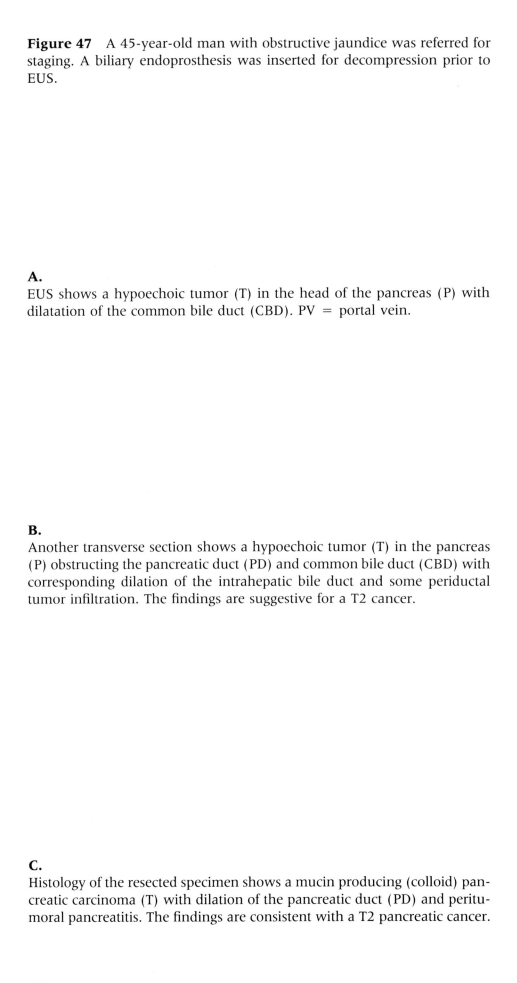

A.
EUS shows a hypoechoic tumor (T) in the head of the pancreas (P) with dilatation of the common bile duct (CBD). PV = portal vein.

B.
Another transverse section shows a hypoechoic tumor (T) in the pancreas (P) obstructing the pancreatic duct (PD) and common bile duct (CBD) with corresponding dilation of the intrahepatic bile duct and some periductal tumor infiltration. The findings are suggestive for a T2 cancer.

C.
Histology of the resected specimen shows a mucin producing (colloid) pancreatic carcinoma (T) with dilation of the pancreatic duct (PD) and peritumoral pancreatitis. The findings are consistent with a T2 pancreatic cancer.

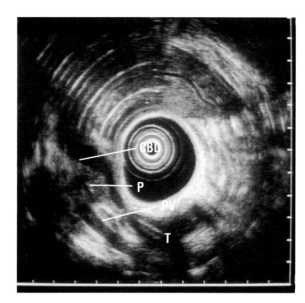

A.

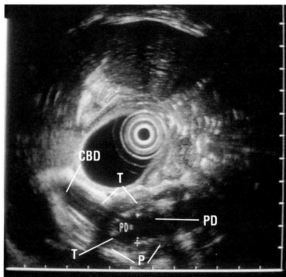

B.

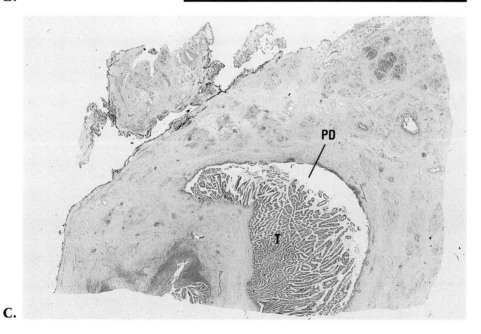

C.

Figure 48 A 70-year-old man with a double duct lesion on ERCP was referred for EUS. An extensive tumor mass in the pancreatic head was found that was extremely suspicious of deep retroperitoneal penetration.

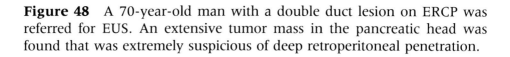

A.
EUS shows a hypoechoic pancreatic carcinoma (T) with retroperitoneal extension to the aorta (AO) and vena cava (VC).

B.
Another transverse section shows an extensive hypoechoic tumor (T) with dilation of the common bile duct (CBD) and pancreatic duct (PD) and penetration (arrow) into the portal vein (PV) at the junction with the superior mesenteric vein (SMV). Note the dilation of the pancreatic duct (PD). EN = biliary endoprosthesis.

C.
CT shows a tumor mass (T) between the vena cava (VC) and the splenoportal confluens (CF). Note the narrowing (arrows) of splenoportal confluens and the close proximity of the tumor to the superior mesenteric artery (SMA). GB = gallbladder, AO = aorta.

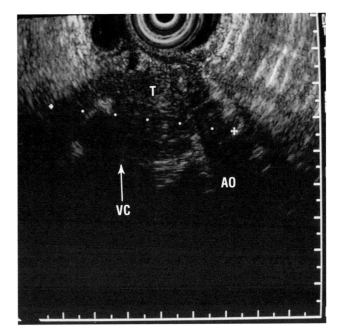

A.

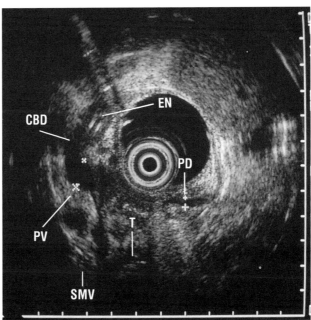

B.

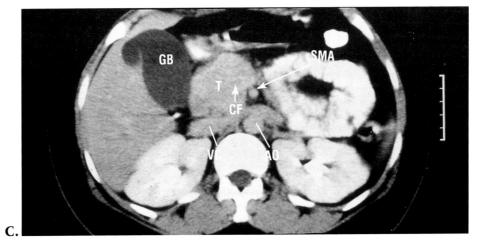

C.

Figure 49 In a 71-year-old woman, a tumor mass was found on CT. Biliary stenting was performed because of obstructive jaundice.

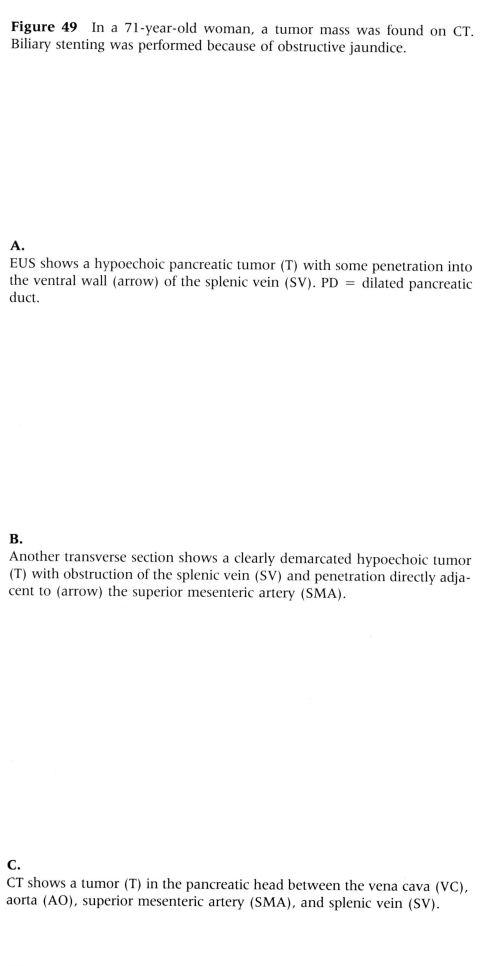

A.
EUS shows a hypoechoic pancreatic tumor (T) with some penetration into the ventral wall (arrow) of the splenic vein (SV). PD = dilated pancreatic duct.

B.
Another transverse section shows a clearly demarcated hypoechoic tumor (T) with obstruction of the splenic vein (SV) and penetration directly adjacent to (arrow) the superior mesenteric artery (SMA).

C.
CT shows a tumor (T) in the pancreatic head between the vena cava (VC), aorta (AO), superior mesenteric artery (SMA), and splenic vein (SV).

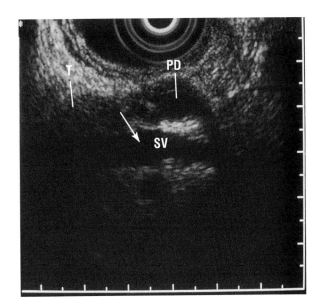

A.

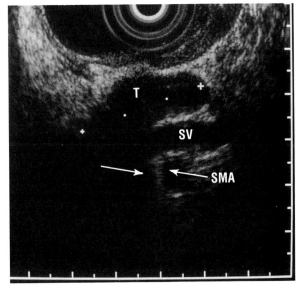

B.

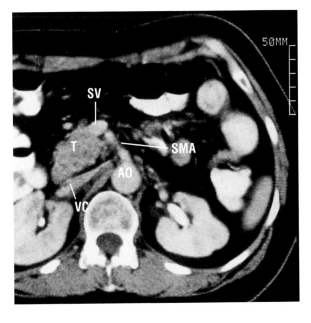

C.

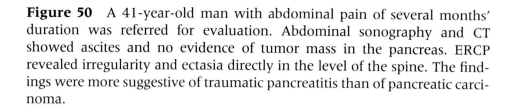

Figure 50 A 41-year-old man with abdominal pain of several months' duration was referred for evaluation. Abdominal sonography and CT showed ascites and no evidence of tumor mass in the pancreas. ERCP revealed irregularity and ectasia directly in the level of the spine. The findings were more suggestive of traumatic pancreatitis than of pancreatic carcinoma.

A.
EUS shows a hypoechoic tumor (T) in the body of the pancreas with prestenotic dilatation of the pancreatic duct (PD), obstruction (arrows) of the splenic vein (SV), and ascites in the bursa omentalis (AS).

B.
Another transverse section shows fundic varices (VAR) due to segmental portal hypertension.

C.
ERCP shows narrowing of Wirsung's duct (PD) in the body of the pancreas at the level of the spine with some irregularity of the side branches. The patient died shortly (2 months) after explorative laparotomy because of metastatic pancreatic cancer.

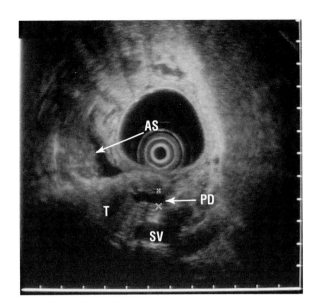

A.

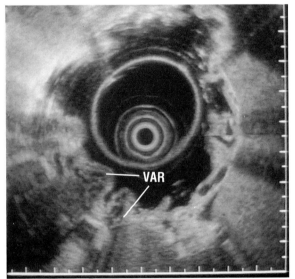

B.

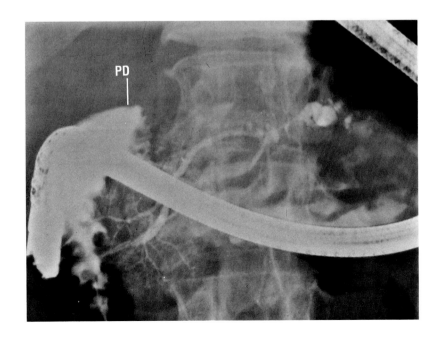

C.

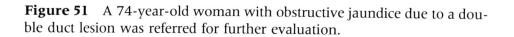

Figure 51 A 74-year-old woman with obstructive jaundice due to a double duct lesion was referred for further evaluation.

A.
EUS shows an extensive hypoechoic tumor (T) with an obstruction of the portal vein (PV) adjacent to the splenoportal confluence. CBD = common bile duct, EN = biliary endoprosthesis.

B.
Another transverse section shows a hypoechoic tumor (T) with obstruction of the portal vein (PV). Note the narrowing of part of the portal vein due to tumor infiltration (arrows). CBD = common bile duct.

C.
Splenoportography shows an obstruction of the splenoportal junction (arrows). PV = extrahepatic portal vein, SV = splenic vein, EN = biliary endoprosthesis, CAT = angiography catheter, SP = spleen, PV = portal vein.

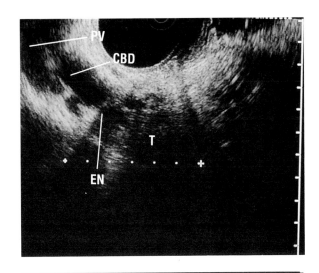

A.

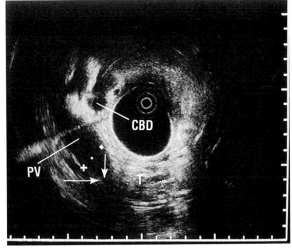

B.

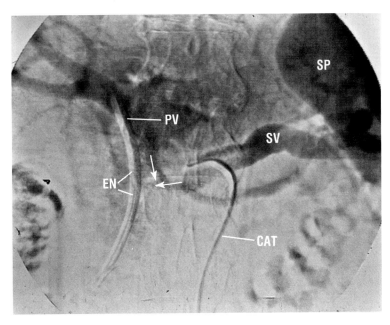

C.

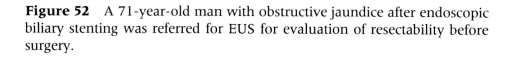

Figure 52 A 71-year-old man with obstructive jaundice after endoscopic biliary stenting was referred for EUS for evaluation of resectability before surgery.

A.

EUS shows a polypoid intraductal tumor (T) in the intrapancreatic portion of the common bile duct (CBD) with prestenotic dilation and a biliary endoprosthesis (EN). The findings are consistent with a T2 common bile duct cancer.

B.

CT shows an echogenic structure in the pancreas adjacent to the duodenum due to an inserted biliary endoprosthesis (EN), without visualization of the primary lesion.

C.

Histology shows a polypoid intraductal carcinoma (T) of the common bile duct without penetration through the muscularis propria (MP) consistent with a T1 common bile duct cancer. P = pancreas.

142

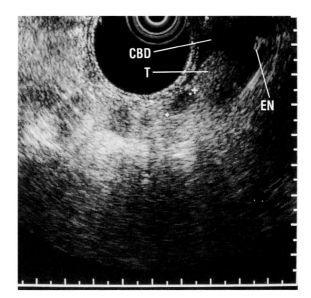

A.

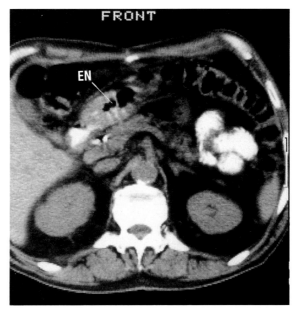

B.

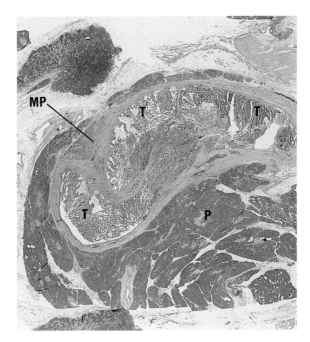

C.

Figure 53 A 71-year-old man with distal common bile duct obstruction due to cholangiocarcinoma was referred for EUS.

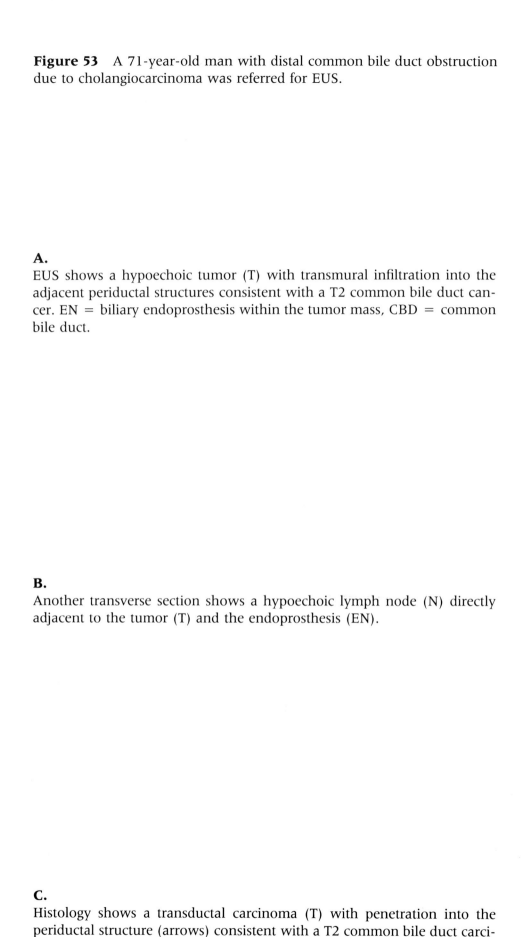

A.
EUS shows a hypoechoic tumor (T) with transmural infiltration into the adjacent periductal structures consistent with a T2 common bile duct cancer. EN = biliary endoprosthesis within the tumor mass, CBD = common bile duct.

B.
Another transverse section shows a hypoechoic lymph node (N) directly adjacent to the tumor (T) and the endoprosthesis (EN).

C.
Histology shows a transductal carcinoma (T) with penetration into the periductal structure (arrows) consistent with a T2 common bile duct carcinoma. P = pancreas with some peritumoral pancreatitis.

144

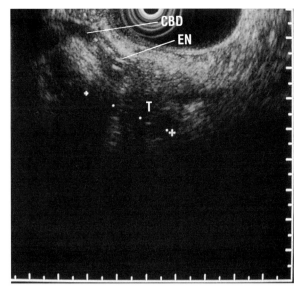

A.

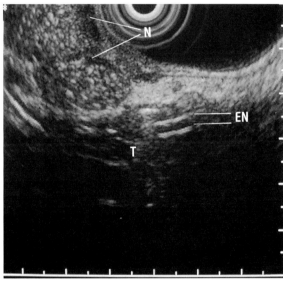

B.

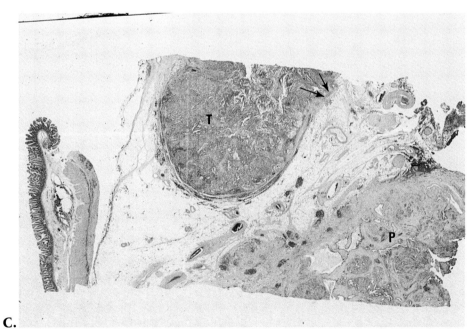

C.

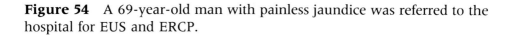

Figure 54 A 69-year-old man with painless jaundice was referred to the hospital for EUS and ERCP.

A.
EUS shows a transductal hypoechoic tumor (T) with prestenotic dilatation of the common bile duct (CBD). The tumor shows a close proximity to the portal vein (PV) but with no evidence of infiltration into the vessel wall. There is still some hypoechoic pattern between the tumor and the portal vein (arrows).

B.
Another transverse section shows some polypoid tumor (arrows) in the wall of the common bile duct (CBD) and the intrapancreatic extent of the tumor (T). P = pancreas, PV = portal vein, SMV = superior mesenteric vein, SV = splenic vein.

C.
ERCP shows an obstruction (arrows) of the intrapancreatic common bile duct (CBD) with prestenotic dilatation but with no evidence of involvement of the pancreatic duct (PD).

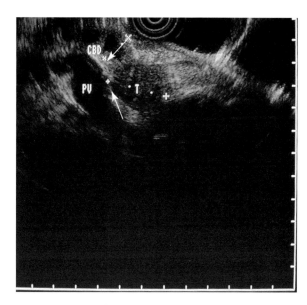

A.

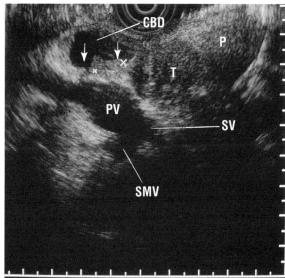

B.

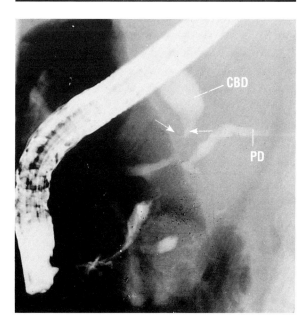

C.

Figure 55   A 68-year-old man presented with obstructive jaundice without gallstone disease. For decompression of the biliary tract, endoscopic drainage was performed. Clinical staging with EUS was performed before surgery.

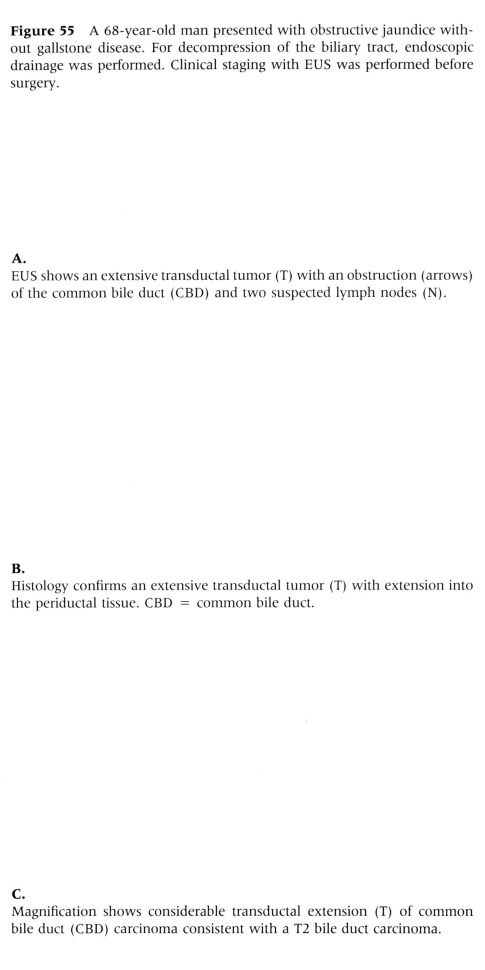

A.
EUS shows an extensive transductal tumor (T) with an obstruction (arrows) of the common bile duct (CBD) and two suspected lymph nodes (N).

B.
Histology confirms an extensive transductal tumor (T) with extension into the periductal tissue. CBD = common bile duct.

C.
Magnification shows considerable transductal extension (T) of common bile duct (CBD) carcinoma consistent with a T2 bile duct carcinoma.

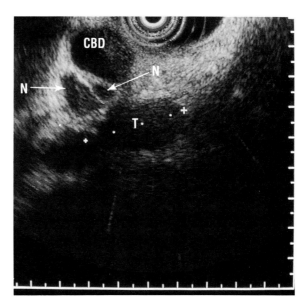

A.

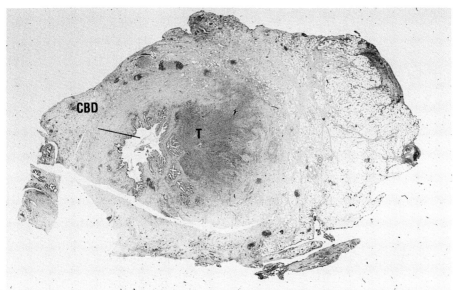

B.

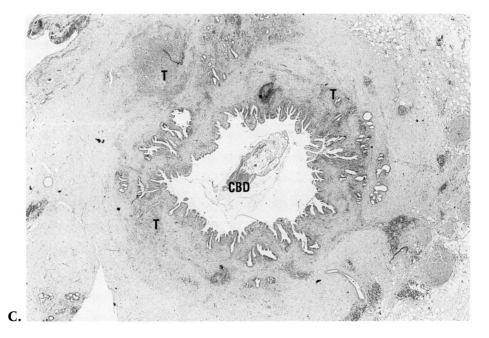

C.

Figure 56 A 70-year-old woman with cholestiasis but without evidence of icterus was referred for evaluation. ERCP revealed an obstruction in the intrapancreatic common bile duct.

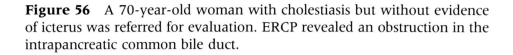

A.
EUS shows a hypoechoic transductal common bile duct carcinoma (T) penetrating (arrows) into the pancreas with an adjacent lymph node (N). PD = pancreatic duct.

B.
Another cross section shows the tumor (T) with deep penetration (arrows) into the adjacent pancreatic parenchyma (P), the pancreatic duct (PD), and the splenoportal junction strongly suspicious of T3 cancer. SV = splenic vein, N = lymph node adjacent to tumor.

C.
ERCP shows an intrapancreatic tumor (arrows) of the common bile duct (CBD) with prestenotic dilation of the extra- and intrahepatic bile duct. Note some dilatation of the pancreatic duct (PD) adjacent to the tumor. Histology of the resected specimen confirmed the EUS diagnosis concerning the tumor infiltration into the splenoportal junction. CHD = common hepatic duct.

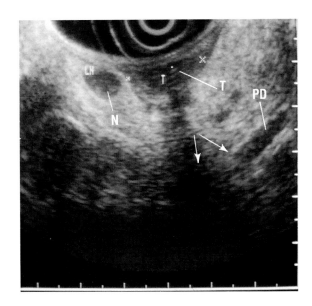

A.

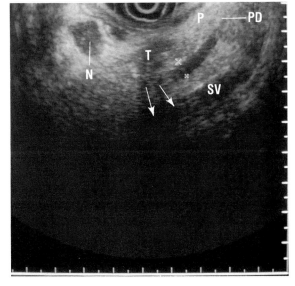

B.

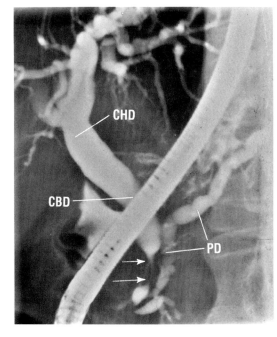

C.

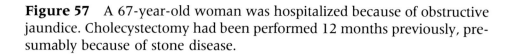

Figure 57 A 67-year-old woman was hospitalized because of obstructive jaundice. Cholecystectomy had been performed 12 months previously, presumably because of stone disease.

A.
EUS shows a large intraductal tumor (T) in the extremely dilated common hepatic duct (HD) with a nondilated common bile duct (CBD) and normal portal vein (PV). L = liver.

B.
Another transverse section shows the tumor (T) extending into the bifurcation (arrows) and transductal invasion. Note the dilated common hepatic ducts (CHD). The findings are consistent with a T2 Klatskin tumor. EN = endoprosthesis, L = liver, CBD = common bile duct.

C.
ERCP shows an extremely dilated common hepatic duct (CHD) with some filling defects due to an extensive polypoid tumor (T). CBD = common bile duct.

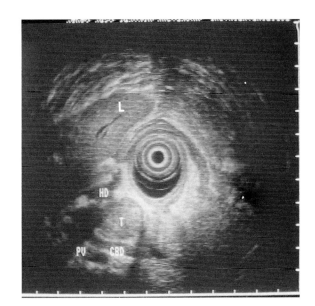

A.

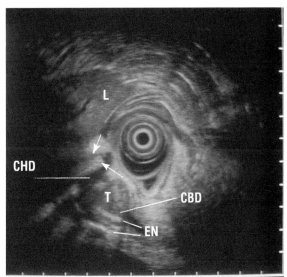

B.

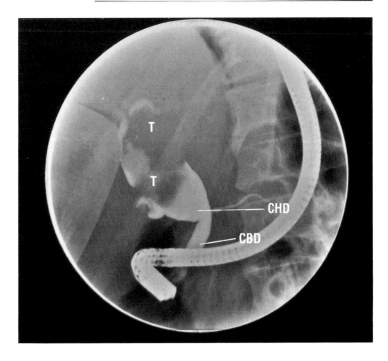

C.

Figure 58 In a 31-year-old man with obstructive jaundice due to a bifurcation tumor, EUS was performed prior to surgery. A biliary endoprosthesis was inserted for decompression.

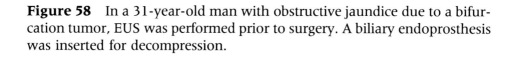

A.
EUS shows a hypoechoic tumor (T) at the bifurcation of the hepatic ducts and a satellite tumor (arrows) next to an inserted endoprosthesis (EN) some distance from the primary tumor adjacent to the intrahepatic portal veins (PV). L = liver.

B.
Another transverse section shows a tumor (T) directly adjacent to the endoprosthesis (EN) at the bifurcation with some transductal invasion into the periductal connective tissue. The findings are strongly suspicious of T2 Klatskin tumor.

C.
Histology shows a cholangiocarcinoma (T) at the bifurcation of the hepatic ducts (HD) consistent with a T2 Klatskin tumor. L = liver parenchyma.

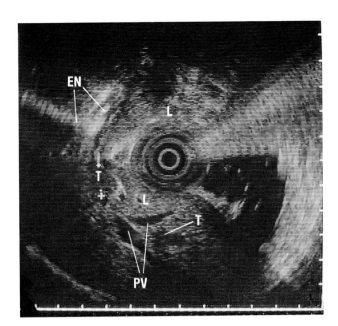

A.

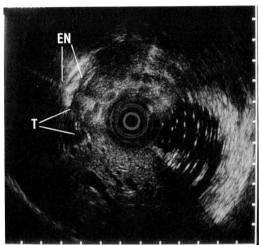

B.

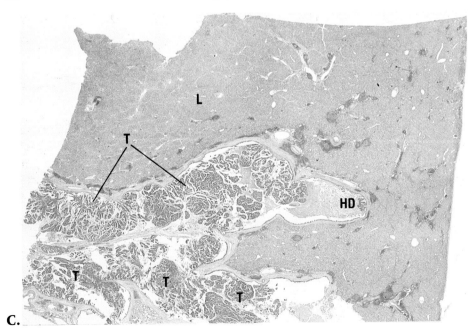

C.

Figure 59 A 62-year-old woman was hospitalized because of obstructive jaundice without stone disease. Sclerosing cholangitis associated with a bifurcation tumor was found on ERCP.

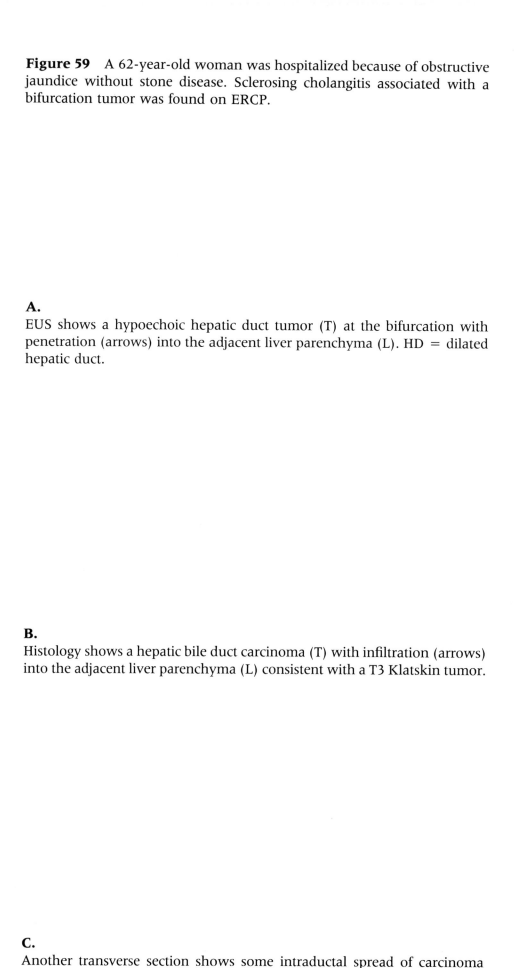

A.
EUS shows a hypoechoic hepatic duct tumor (T) at the bifurcation with penetration (arrows) into the adjacent liver parenchyma (L). HD = dilated hepatic duct.

B.
Histology shows a hepatic bile duct carcinoma (T) with infiltration (arrows) into the adjacent liver parenchyma (L) consistent with a T3 Klatskin tumor.

C.
Another transverse section shows some intraductal spread of carcinoma (T) (multifocal). L = liver parenchyma.

156

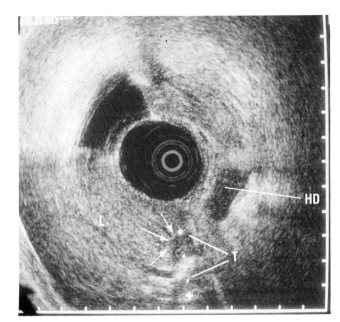

A.

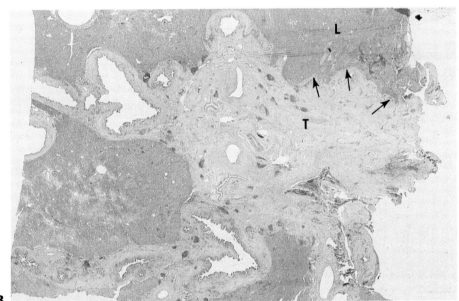

B.

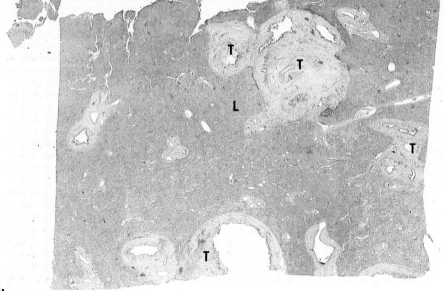

C.

Figure 60 A 58-year-old man with recurrent jaundice for a year was admitted to the hospital. After preoperative staging with EUS and ERCP, hemihepatectomy was performed.

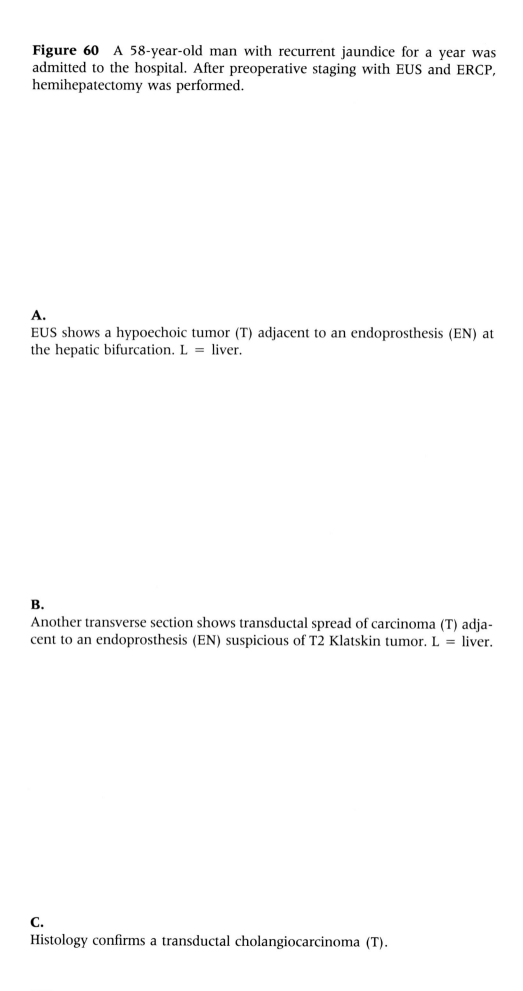

A.
EUS shows a hypoechoic tumor (T) adjacent to an endoprosthesis (EN) at the hepatic bifurcation. L = liver.

B.
Another transverse section shows transductal spread of carcinoma (T) adjacent to an endoprosthesis (EN) suspicious of T2 Klatskin tumor. L = liver.

C.
Histology confirms a transductal cholangiocarcinoma (T).

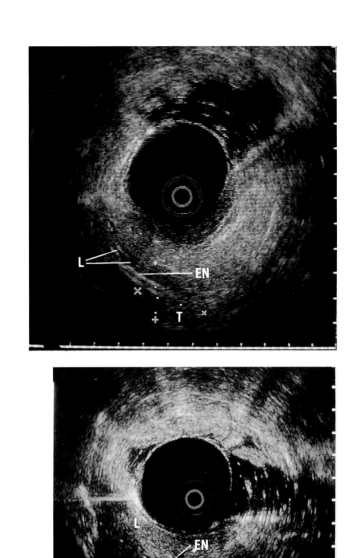

A.

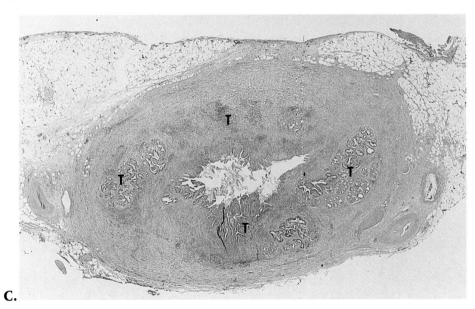

B.

C.

Figure 61 A 59-year-old man with no history of liver and gallstone disease was hospitalized because of obstructive jaundice. ERCP and EUS performed preoperatively revealed a tumor in the proximal bile duct and its bifurcation.

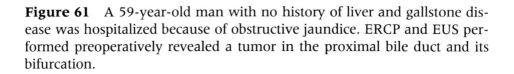

A.
EUS shows a hypoechoic tumor (T) adjacent to the liver hilum (L) with transductal spread and an metastatic involved lymph node (N). EN = biliary endoprosthesis.

B.
ERCP shows a narrowed common hepatic duct (arrows) with prestenotic dilation of intra- and extrahepatic bile ducts (HD). PD = pancreatic duct, CBD = common bile duct.

C.
Histology shows a polypoid transductal cholangiocarcinoma (T) of the common hepatic duct (HD).

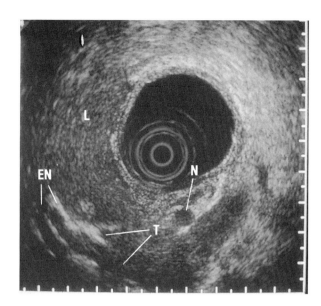

A.

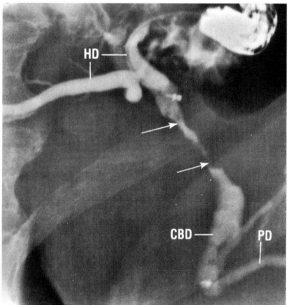

B.

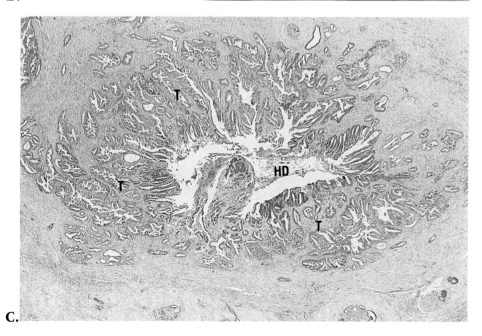

C.

Figure 62 A 68-year-old man with painless obstructive jaundice was referred for evaluation.

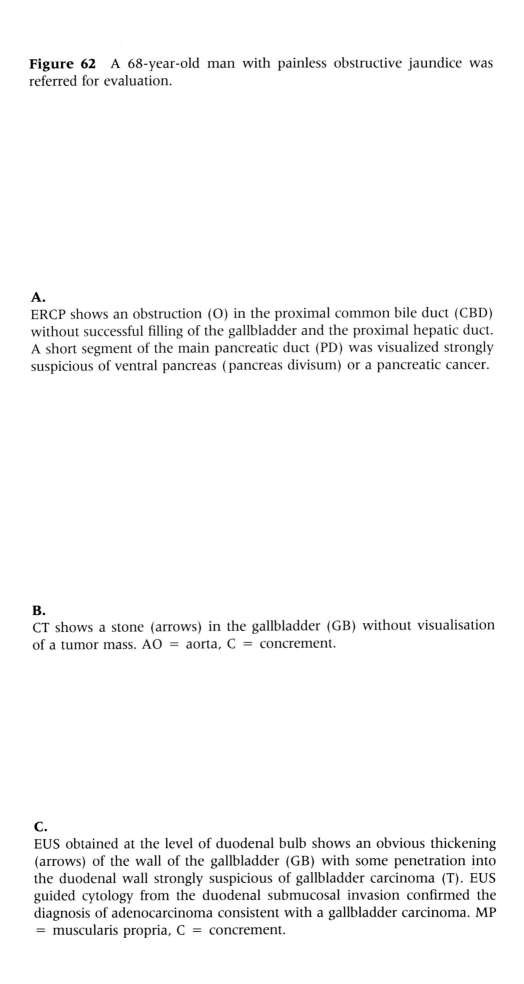

A.
ERCP shows an obstruction (O) in the proximal common bile duct (CBD) without successful filling of the gallbladder and the proximal hepatic duct. A short segment of the main pancreatic duct (PD) was visualized strongly suspicious of ventral pancreas (pancreas divisum) or a pancreatic cancer.

B.
CT shows a stone (arrows) in the gallbladder (GB) without visualisation of a tumor mass. AO = aorta, C = concrement.

C.
EUS obtained at the level of duodenal bulb shows an obvious thickening (arrows) of the wall of the gallbladder (GB) with some penetration into the duodenal wall strongly suspicious of gallbladder carcinoma (T). EUS guided cytology from the duodenal submucosal invasion confirmed the diagnosis of adenocarcinoma consistent with a gallbladder carcinoma. MP = muscularis propria, C = concrement.

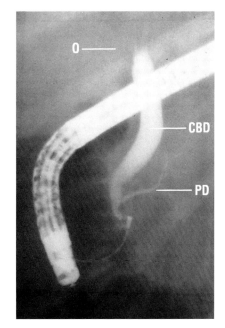

A.

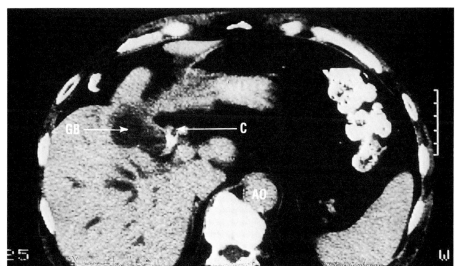

B.

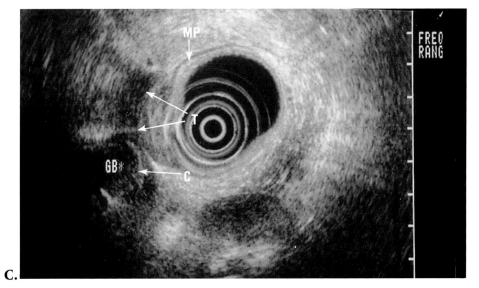

C.

Figure 63

A.
A rigid Aloka transrectal ultrasonic instrument (ASU-57) with an echo-probe (E) (diameter 15 mm, mechanical radial scanner) fixed at the tip of a rigid shaft (length 12 cm) and a water channel (CH) for filling the balloon with water (WB).

B.
A flexible Aloka ultrasonic prototype (ASU-59) with a small echoprobe (E) (diameter 10 mm, mechanic radial scanner) fixed at the tip of a flexible nonoptic shaft (length 65 cm). CH = water channel.

C.
A rigid Aloka transrectal ultrasonic instrument with a linear-array probe (E) fixed beyond the tip (180° linear-array imaging).

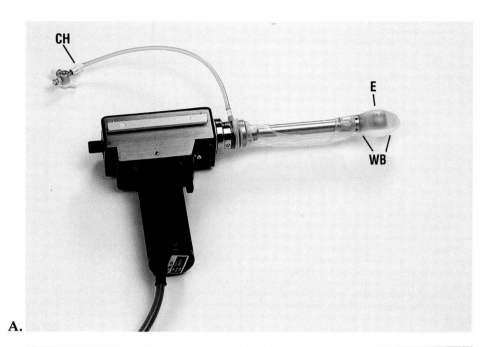

A.

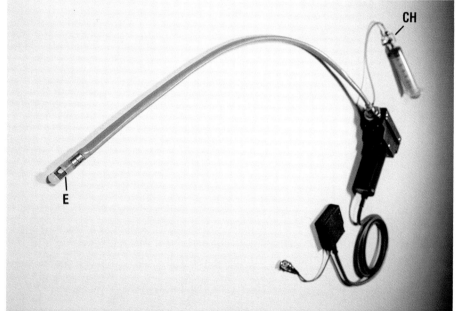

B.

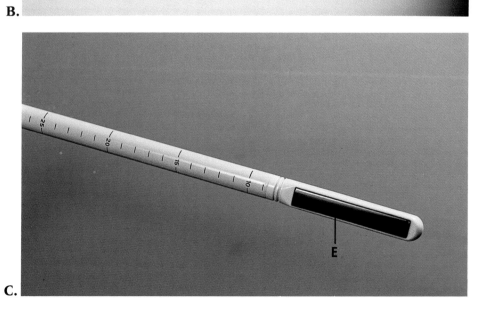

C.

Figure 64

A.

An Olympus echoendoscopic EUM3 with a biopsy forceps (BF) passing through the instrumental channel. Note the echoprobe is attached proximally to the side-viewing optics and the biopsy channel distally to the echoprobe. E = echoprobe.

B.

A prototype Olympus echocoloscope (XCF-UM*) without the possibility for covering the echoprobe (E) with a balloon. Note the echoprobe is attached parallel to the biopsy channel and beyond the optics. CH = working channel, O = optics.

C.

A commercially available Olympus echocolonoscope (XCF-UM2) which can be covered with a balloon for producing an acoustic window. Note the echoprobe is attached parallel to the biopsy channel and beyond the optics. E = echoprobe, CH = working channel, O = optics.

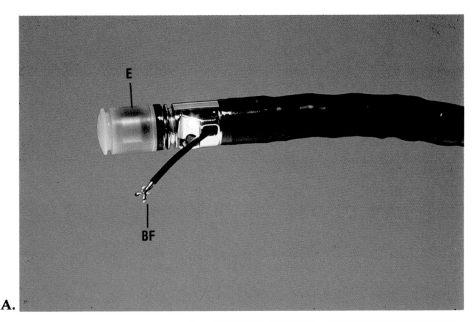

A.

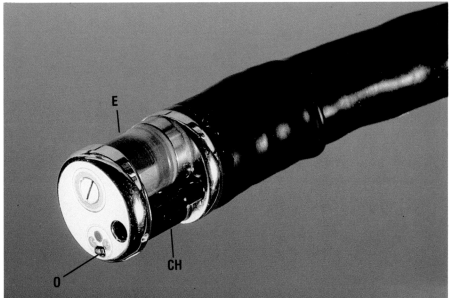

B.

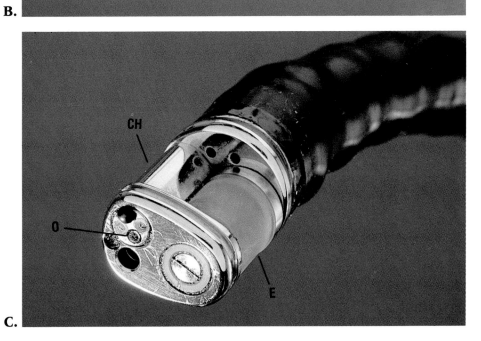

C.

Figure 65 In a 67-year-old man with rectal blood loss a rectal carcinoma was found endoscopically.

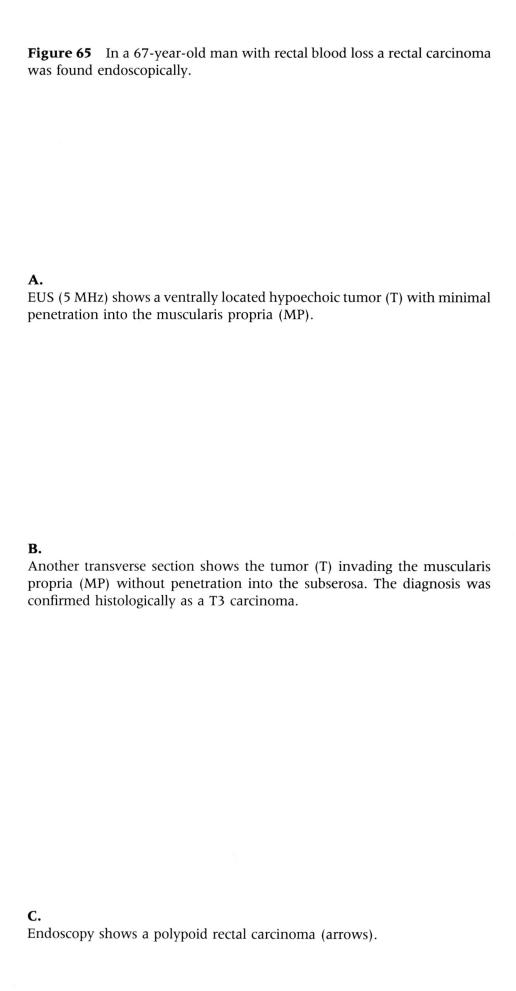

A.
EUS (5 MHz) shows a ventrally located hypoechoic tumor (T) with minimal penetration into the muscularis propria (MP).

B.
Another transverse section shows the tumor (T) invading the muscularis propria (MP) without penetration into the subserosa. The diagnosis was confirmed histologically as a T3 carcinoma.

C.
Endoscopy shows a polypoid rectal carcinoma (arrows).

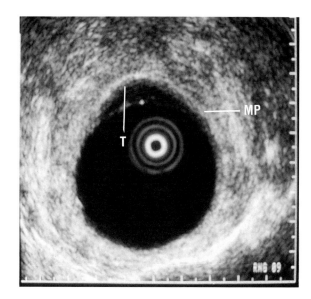

A.

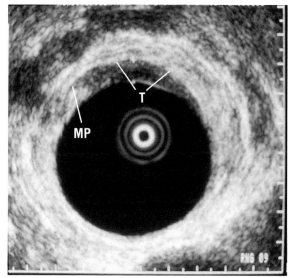

B.

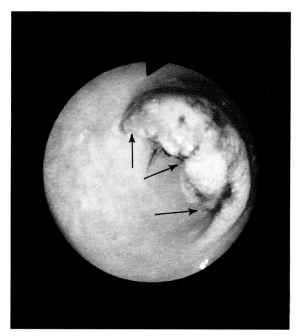

C.

Figure 66 A 62-year-old woman with a rectal carcinoma was referred for EUS.

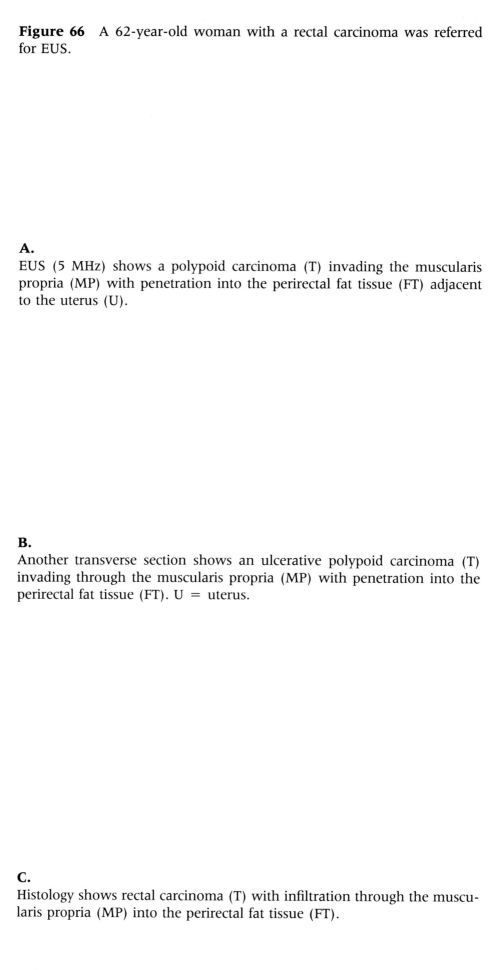

A.
EUS (5 MHz) shows a polypoid carcinoma (T) invading the muscularis propria (MP) with penetration into the perirectal fat tissue (FT) adjacent to the uterus (U).

B.
Another transverse section shows an ulcerative polypoid carcinoma (T) invading through the muscularis propria (MP) with penetration into the perirectal fat tissue (FT). U = uterus.

C.
Histology shows rectal carcinoma (T) with infiltration through the muscularis propria (MP) into the perirectal fat tissue (FT).

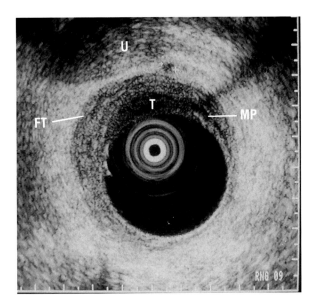

A.

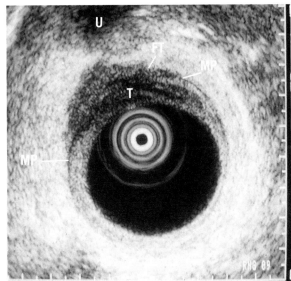

B.

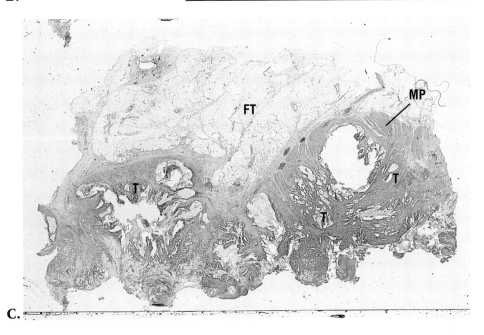

C.

Figure 67 An 81-year-old woman with rectal carcinoma was referred for staging.

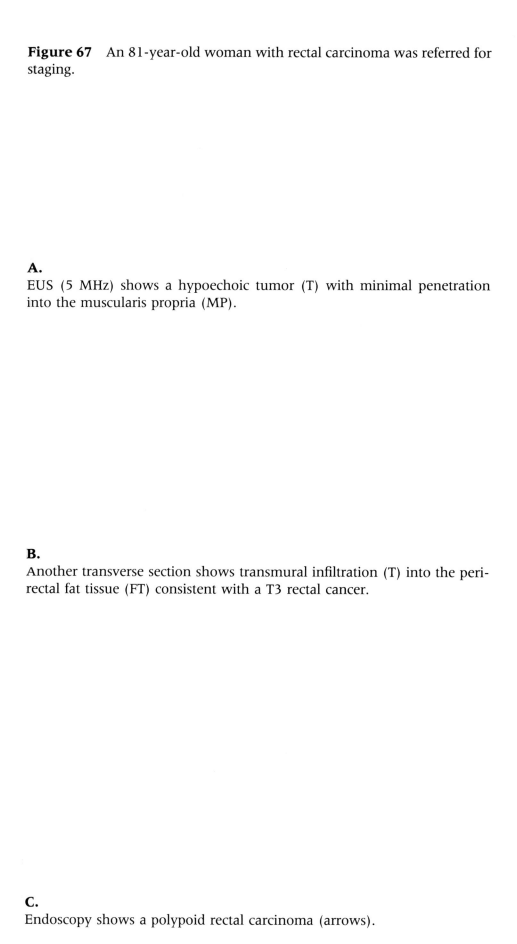

A.
EUS (5 MHz) shows a hypoechoic tumor (T) with minimal penetration into the muscularis propria (MP).

B.
Another transverse section shows transmural infiltration (T) into the perirectal fat tissue (FT) consistent with a T3 rectal cancer.

C.
Endoscopy shows a polypoid rectal carcinoma (arrows).

A.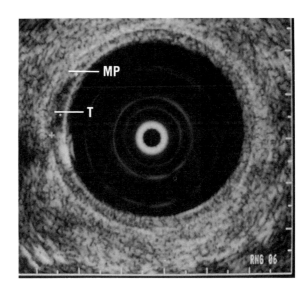

B.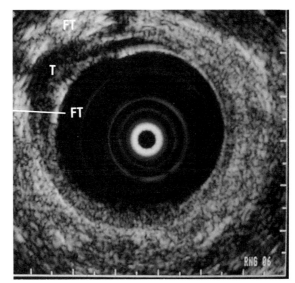

C.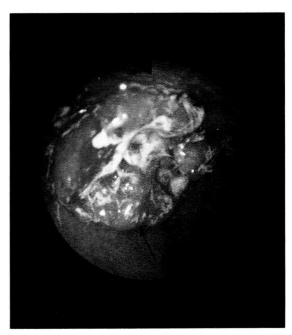

Figure 68 A 60-year-old man with rectal blood loss due to a rectal carcinoma was referred for staging.

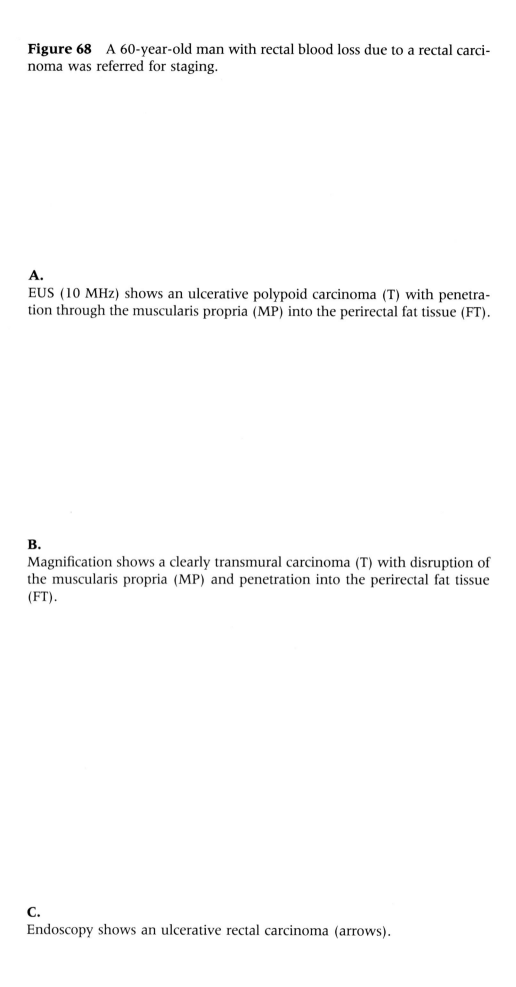

A.
EUS (10 MHz) shows an ulcerative polypoid carcinoma (T) with penetration through the muscularis propria (MP) into the perirectal fat tissue (FT).

B.
Magnification shows a clearly transmural carcinoma (T) with disruption of the muscularis propria (MP) and penetration into the perirectal fat tissue (FT).

C.
Endoscopy shows an ulcerative rectal carcinoma (arrows).

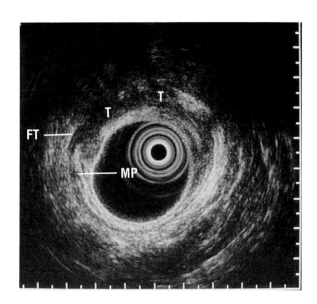

A.

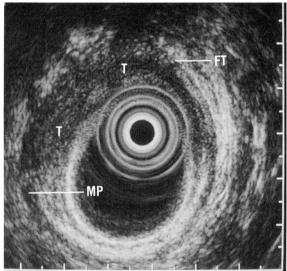

B.

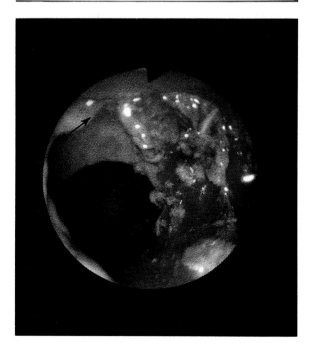

C.

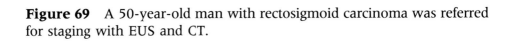

Figure 69 A 50-year-old man with rectosigmoid carcinoma was referred for staging with EUS and CT.

A.

EUS obtained with an echocolonoscope (7.5 MHz) shows a hypoechoic tumor mass (T) with penetration into the muscularis propria (MP). RV = reverberation phenomenon due to the biopsy channel.

B.

Another cross section shows an ulcerative (U) tumor with polypoid margins (arrows). Note the tumor penetration into the perirectal fat tissue (FT) and the total disruption of the muscularis propria adjacent to the tumor (arrowheads).

C.

Corresponding CT shows the wall thickening (T) at the rectosigmoid junction. Note an ulcer (U) with some polypoid margins (arrows).

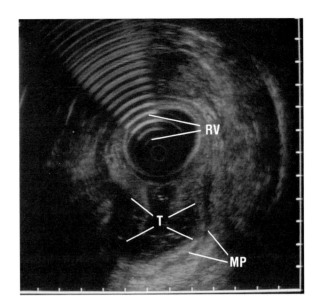

A.

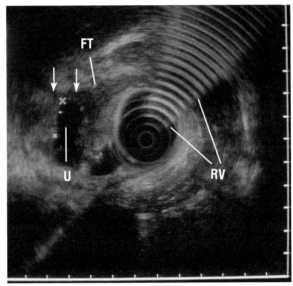

B.

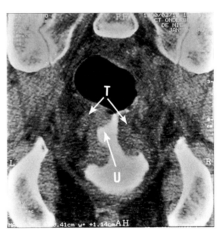

C.

Figure 70 In a 56-year-old man who had undergone radical surgery for cardiac carcinoma 18 months previously, a polypoid bulging lesion at the anastomosis was found radiographically. Endoscopy revealed a stenosis with smooth mucosa. After endoscopic dilatation, EUS was performed because endoscopic biopsies were negative for carcinoma.

A.
EUS shows a semicircular transmural hypoechoic tumor (T) at the left side with deep penetration to the adjacent metallic clips (C) of the esophagogastric anastomosis. The findings are consistent with a recurrent T3 cancer.

B.
Another transverse section shows metastatic lymph nodes (N) adjacent to the carcinomatous infiltration (T). C = metallic clips.

C.
Barium meal shows a double contour (arrows) adjacent to the anastomosis strongly suspicious of recurrent carcinoma.

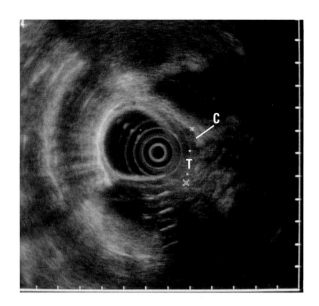

A.

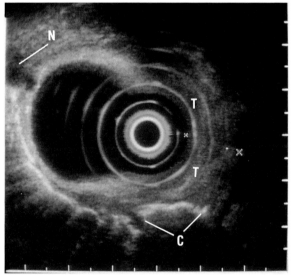

B.

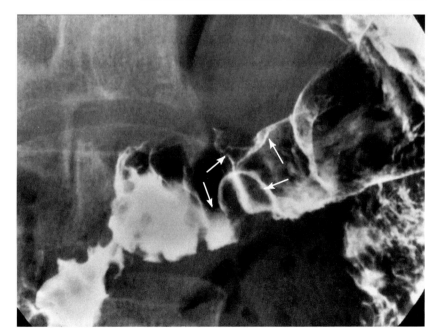

C.

Figure 71 A 66-year-old man underwent a Whipple procedure for a pancreatic carcinoma. Preoperative and follow-up EUS were performed.

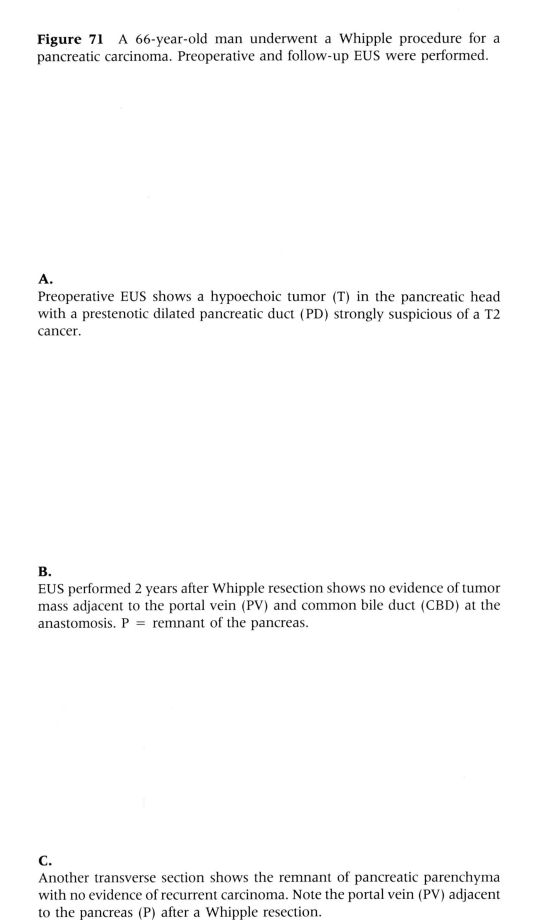

A.
Preoperative EUS shows a hypoechoic tumor (T) in the pancreatic head with a prestenotic dilated pancreatic duct (PD) strongly suspicious of a T2 cancer.

B.
EUS performed 2 years after Whipple resection shows no evidence of tumor mass adjacent to the portal vein (PV) and common bile duct (CBD) at the anastomosis. P = remnant of the pancreas.

C.
Another transverse section shows the remnant of pancreatic parenchyma with no evidence of recurrent carcinoma. Note the portal vein (PV) adjacent to the pancreas (P) after a Whipple resection.

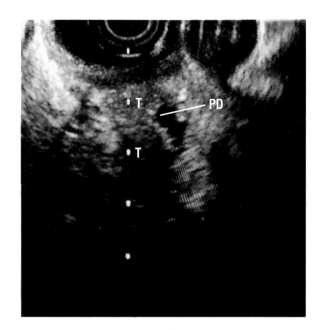

A.

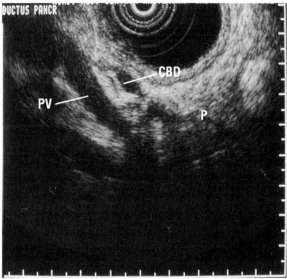

B.

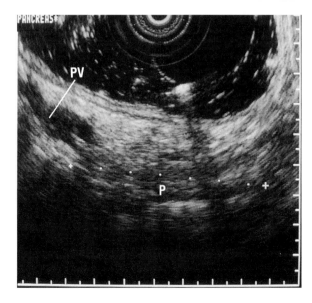

C.

Figure 72 A 64-year-old man with obstructive jaundice suspicious of pancreatic carcinoma was hospitalized for surgery. Preoperative and follow-up EUS were performed.

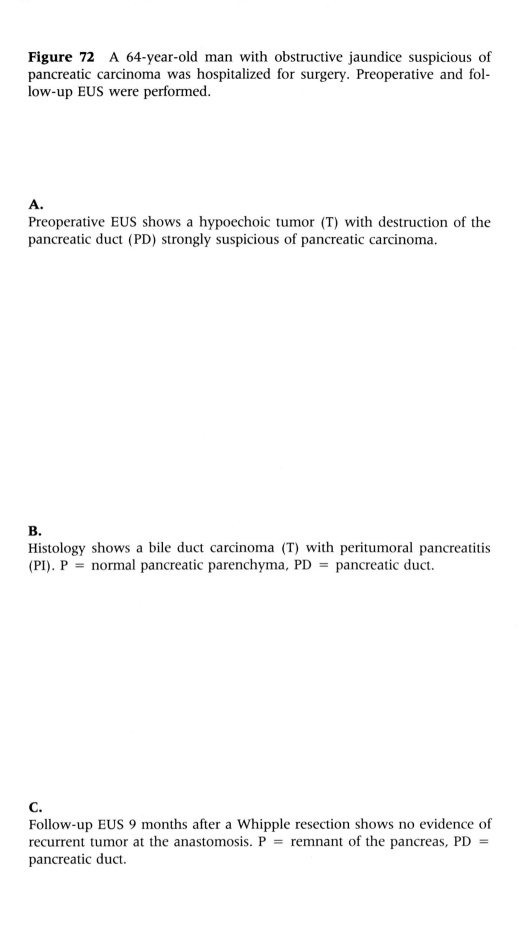

A.
Preoperative EUS shows a hypoechoic tumor (T) with destruction of the pancreatic duct (PD) strongly suspicious of pancreatic carcinoma.

B.
Histology shows a bile duct carcinoma (T) with peritumoral pancreatitis (PI). P = normal pancreatic parenchyma, PD = pancreatic duct.

C.
Follow-up EUS 9 months after a Whipple resection shows no evidence of recurrent tumor at the anastomosis. P = remnant of the pancreas, PD = pancreatic duct.

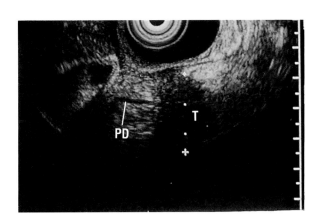

A.

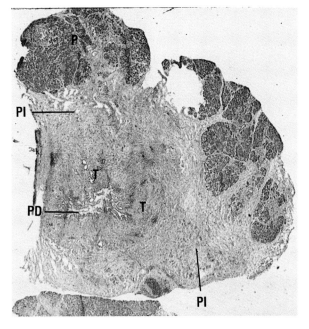

B.

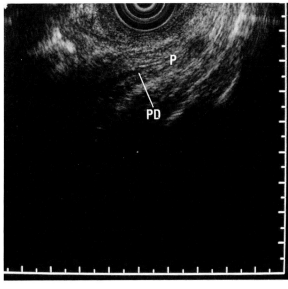

C.

Figure 73 In a 74-year-old man who had previously undergone low anterior resection for carcinoma, endoscopy and EUS revealed a recurrent carcinoma at the anastomosis.

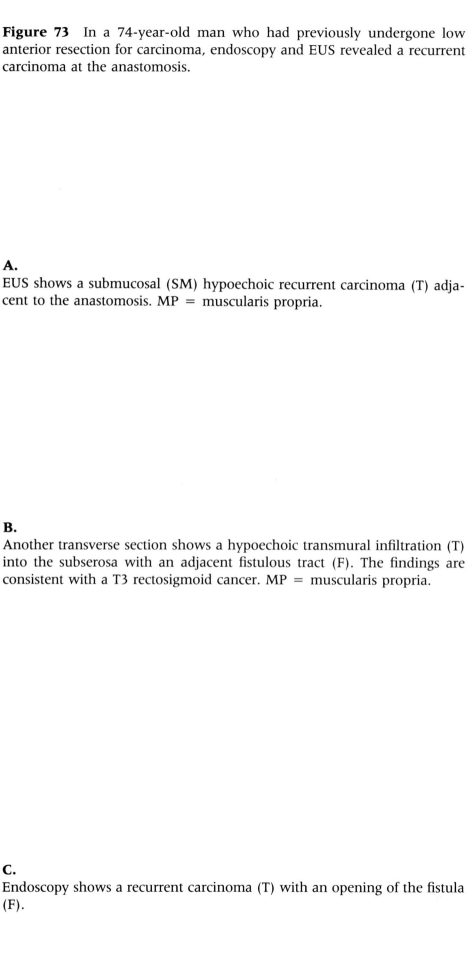

A.
EUS shows a submucosal (SM) hypoechoic recurrent carcinoma (T) adjacent to the anastomosis. MP = muscularis propria.

B.
Another transverse section shows a hypoechoic transmural infiltration (T) into the subserosa with an adjacent fistulous tract (F). The findings are consistent with a T3 rectosigmoid cancer. MP = muscularis propria.

C.
Endoscopy shows a recurrent carcinoma (T) with an opening of the fistula (F).

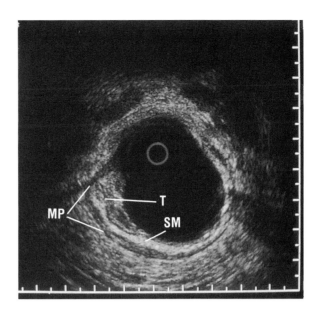

A.

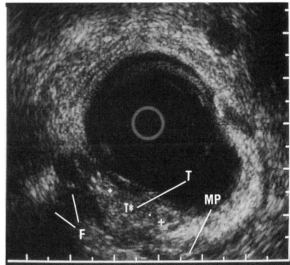

B.

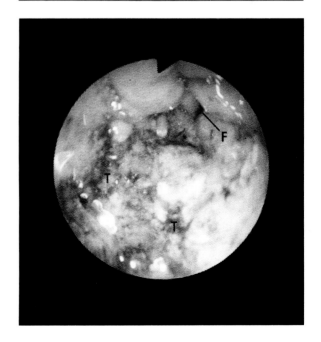

C.

Figure 74 A 77-year-old man with poor medical condition was referred for surgery. EUS was performed prior to laser treatment for the staging of gastric carcinoma.

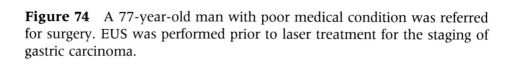

A.
Before laser treatment, EUS shows a hypoechoic intrasubmucosal tumor (T) without penetration into the muscularis propria (MP) consistent with an early gastric carcinoma.

B.
During follow-up over a period of 5 years, EUS shows no change in the depth of infiltration (T) after laser treatment. Note the hyperechoic pattern at the surface due to an ulcerative (U) lesion after laser treatment. MP = muscularis propria.

C.
Endoscopy shows an ulcerative lesion after laser treatment (arrows).

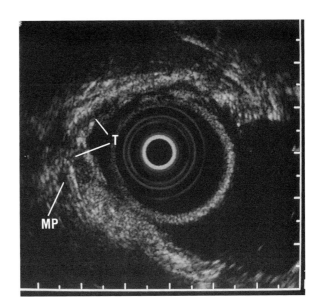

A.

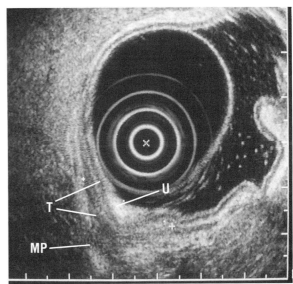

B.

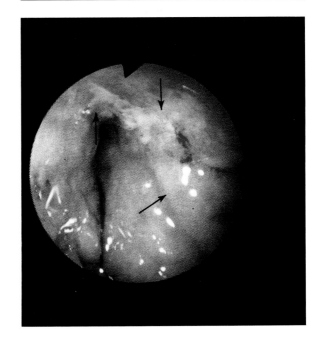

C.

Figure 75 A 66-year-old woman with extensive esophageal carcinoma that proved to be nonresectable at surgery was referred for EUS before and after combined intraluminal (after loading) and external radiotherapy.

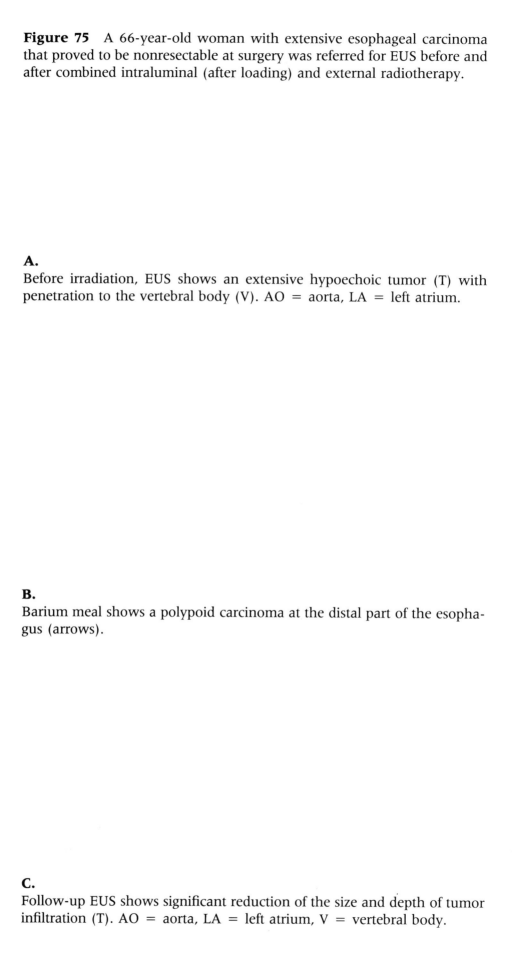

A.
Before irradiation, EUS shows an extensive hypoechoic tumor (T) with penetration to the vertebral body (V). AO = aorta, LA = left atrium.

B.
Barium meal shows a polypoid carcinoma at the distal part of the esophagus (arrows).

C.
Follow-up EUS shows significant reduction of the size and depth of tumor infiltration (T). AO = aorta, LA = left atrium, V = vertebral body.

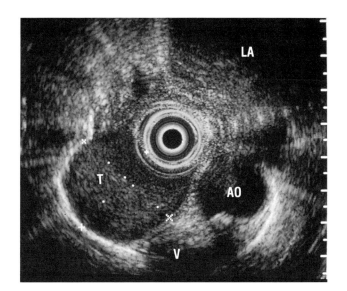

A.

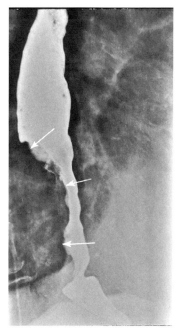

B.

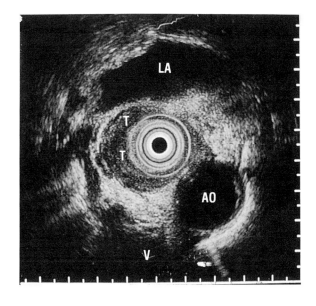

C.

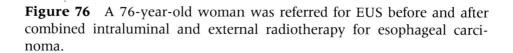

Figure 76 A 76-year-old woman was referred for EUS before and after combined intraluminal and external radiotherapy for esophageal carcinoma.

A.
Before irradiation, EUS shows a transmural hypoechoic exophytic carcinoma (T) with adjacent metastatic lymph nodes (N). The findings are consistent with T3 N1 esophageal cancer nodes. LA = left atrium, AO = aorta.

B.
Follow-up EUS shows reduction of mural infiltration (T). The involved lymph node (N), however, does not show any change in size and echo pattern. AO = aorta, LA = left atrium.

C.
Ten months after irradiation, progression of mural infiltration (T) is demonstrated. The patient died due to carcinomatous spread. Note the increase of tumor thickness as compared to the previous findings. AO = aorta, LA = left atrium.

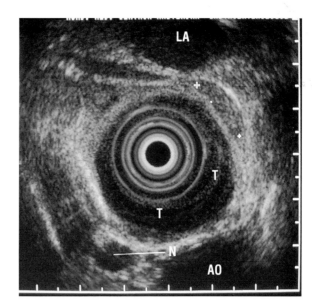

A.

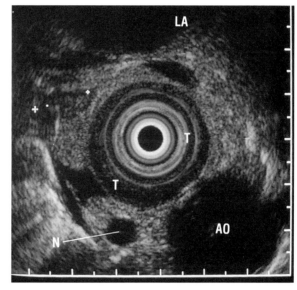

B.

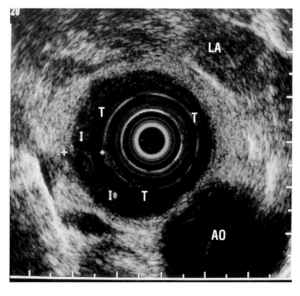

C.

Figure 77 In the following three patients with severe stenotic esophageal carcinoma which could not be passed with EUS instruments, a catheter echoprobe was inserted into the stenotic region.

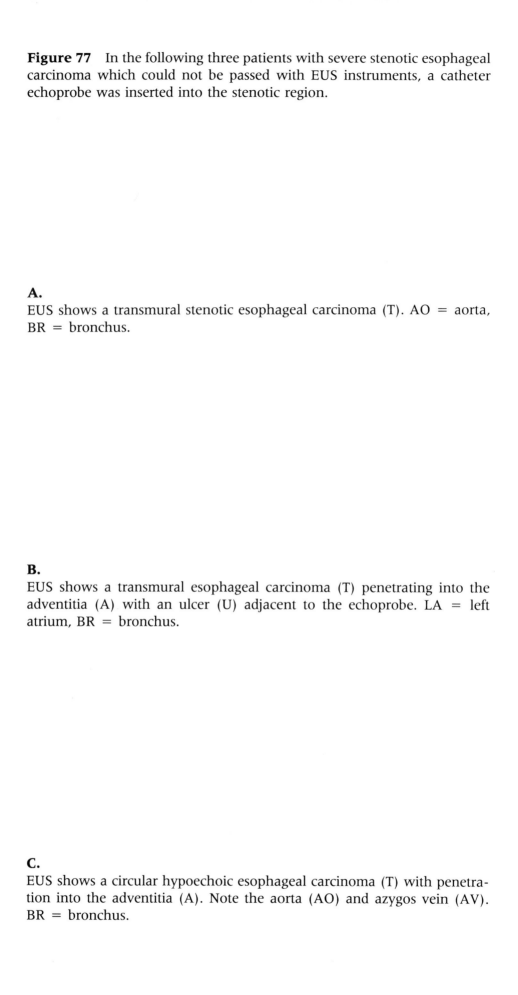

A.
EUS shows a transmural stenotic esophageal carcinoma (T). AO = aorta, BR = bronchus.

B.
EUS shows a transmural esophageal carcinoma (T) penetrating into the adventitia (A) with an ulcer (U) adjacent to the echoprobe. LA = left atrium, BR = bronchus.

C.
EUS shows a circular hypoechoic esophageal carcinoma (T) with penetration into the adventitia (A). Note the aorta (AO) and azygos vein (AV). BR = bronchus.

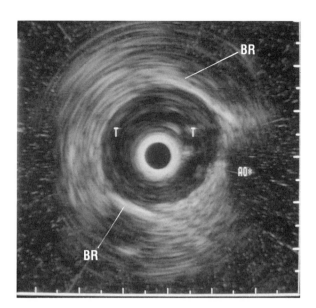

A.

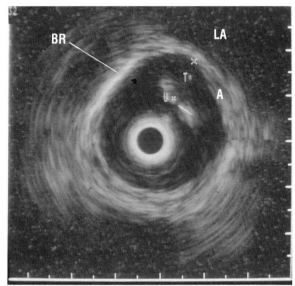

B.

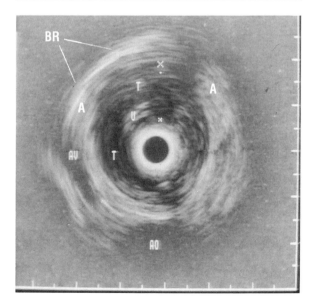

C.

Index